# Contents

| | |
|---|---|
| Acknowledgements | 7 |
| Preface | 9 |
| Part I: Sara's Story | 13 |
| Part II: Facts and Questions | 105 |
| Guilt | 107 |
| Problem Thunderstorm | 108 |
| Explanations | 110 |
| Heredity and Asthma | 111 |
| Games | 112 |
| Pets | 114 |
| Breath Control and Yoga | 115 |
| Relaxation Exercises | 115 |
| What about the Heart and Lungs? | 117 |
| Air Travel | 117 |
| Clothing | 117 |
| The Asthma Attack | 118 |
| Don't Settle for Second Best | 120 |
| Asthma and Allergy | 122 |
| Exercise Asthma | 127 |
| Asthma: All in the Mind? | 131 |
| Steroids | 134 |
| Will My Child grow out of Asthma? | 140 |
| Questions and Answers | 141 |
| Organisations | 151 |
| Glossary | 155 |
| Book List | 168 |
| Index | 169 |

# HELP ME, MUMMY, I CAN'T BREATHE

*HUMAN HORIZONS SERIES*

# HELP ME, MUMMY, I CAN'T BREATHE
## Coping with Childhood Asthma

SUSAN SUTHERLAND

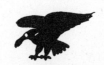

A CONDOR BOOK
SOUVENIR PRESS (E & A) LTD

ISBN 0 285 65035 1 casebound ✓
ISBN 0 285 65036 X paperback

Photoset and printed in Great Britain by
WBC Print Ltd, Bristol

# Acknowledgements

Many people have helped in the preparation of this book. Above all, I should like to thank Hugh Faulkner, OBE, Director of the Asthma Society and Friends of the Asthma Research Council, who has been, quite simply, the linchpin of the whole enterprise. Professor Tony Milner has given invaluable help and found time in his packed schedule to read, advise and encourage, and Dr. A.W. Frankland kindly supplied helpful comments about the problems of wheezy bronchitis and childish wheezing.

My thanks also to the following for willingly providing me with information and photographs: Richard Binfield of Clement Clarke International Ltd; the Canadian High Commission; Dr Fleming Carswell (for his remarkable photograph of the house dust mite); R.C. Colley of Astra Pharmaceuticals; Miss Colquhoun of the Reference Library, Australian High Commission; Embassy of the United States of America; Valerie Evans of Cameron Price Medical Division Ltd; Gill Hilsdon of Fisons Pharmaceuticals; Susan Hughes of Allen & Hanbury Ltd; Leeds City Education Department; the New Zealand High Commission; Mrs L. Gration of Austicks bookshop, Leeds; David Stimpson of Medix Ltd; Westways Riding Stables; and the Aquarium Department of Leeds University.

I am grateful to Churchill Livingstone for permission to quote a passage on wheezy bronchitis from *Asthma in Childhood* by A.D. Milner and to Oxford University Press for allowing me to adapt the list of drugs that appeared in *Asthma: the Facts* by Donald J. Lane and Anthony Storr.

My gratitude and deepest respect must go to Dr R. Mowla for his gift of healing; and my sincere admiration and appreciation to every single member of staff of Leeds General Infirmary, for their capacity to generate such a purposeful and heartening atmosphere. Warmest thanks to Marion Donaldson and Lana Odelle for their early encouragement; thanks, too, to Tessa Harrow, my unflagging editor.

Lastly, I must thank my family—'the team'—for all their love and support.

Susan Sutherland
September, 1986

# Preface

Asthma *kills* up to 1,800 people each year in Great Britain alone. Although as many as ten per cent of the population suffer from asthma at some time or other, perhaps as few as three per cent are actually diagnosed asthmatics. That is to say, their recurrent bouts of coughing and wheezing respond well to asthma medications. The incidence of asthma in childhood is even higher. It is now known that as many as one in seven children suffer some degree of asthma, but because a small number of these have symptoms which are extremely mild or occur infrequently, treatment is not sought. Many other asthmatics, more seriously affected, may have escaped the diagnostician's net altogether and are struggling along on their own, hardly knowing what ails them. There are so many asthma sufferers that it is difficult to understand why this unpleasant condition receives so little attention.

I shall go on to show in this book how my seven-year-old daughter, Sara, herself a chronic asthmatic, was frequently dismissed in the early days of her illness by inexperienced general practitioners, because they could not hear anything wrong with her chest. I myself was regarded as something of a 'nuisance'—a typical neurotic mother.

The correct diagnosis and appropriate medications are paramount in the treatment of asthma. Do not be discouraged by anyone, whoever they are, if you feel that your child might be asthmatic. If your local GP cannot help, ask him to refer you to a chest consultant. If that does not work, take your child to your local hospital's casualty department and ask the casualty officer there to refer your child instead.

Above all, have the confidence to be persistent. Asthmatics and parents of asthmatic children have a much keener awareness of the extent of their problem than a doctor can be expected to acquire during a casual visit to his consulting room. In all probability, the attack will have subsided by this time.

The prelude to an attack may manifest itself in any number of ways, possibly unique to the individual concerned, and is hardly noticeable even to the most objective and highly trained observer. I know now when Sara is going to be ill, although I can hardly tell you how I know; my feelings are compounded from experience and intuition. She is normally an extremely bright and active child, but when an attack threatens, she becomes lethargic and dull, sometimes even dropping off to sleep at the most unexpected times. This could be seen as quite normal behaviour for a small child who has possibly 'tired herself out' with an ordinary day's excitement and activity, but for Sara it is both an unusual occurrence and a warning sign. Although her general appearance at these times may be of good health and her breathing quite normal, should I overlook this break in her usual behaviour pattern and allow her to remain without medication, I would expect her to develop a 'wheeze' within a very short space of time. The medication to which I refer in this instance is Ventolin, a widely used 'bronchodilator'. In Sara's case, I have often found that an attack treated promptly in its very earliest stages can be aborted.

Some asthmatics do not appear to wheeze at all, but have a persistent and exhausting cough. This is usually most apparent, not to mention distressing, during the night. In the early days of Sara's illness, this is how her asthmatic condition first manifested itself. To begin with, it was reasonable to accept the assurances of several doctors that she was suffering from frequent mild virus infections, but it is difficult to receive the reassurance you seek, when large city practices make it virtually impossible to see the same doctor on consecutive visits. In order to build up a clearer picture of what was happening to Sara, I began to keep a diary of her illness, to guard against the casual dismissals which we had received at first. I do not necessarily blame tired, sometimes overworked, and very human doctors, who all face exactly the same day-to-day irritations and problems as the rest of us, but I do believe that it is essential for the patient or her parent to be well prepared, even to the extent of compiling a 'check-list' of worries, rather than trust to memory. In this way, you can make the best use of the short time spent with the doctor.

Research into the treatment and control of asthma has made great strides in the past twenty years. At one time, frequent unpleasant injections and many hospital admissions could be expected. Nowadays most medicines are inhaled, so allowing the asthmatic to live a normal life. Never be frightened to accept that your child has asthma; by not accepting this fact, you will be denying the child freedom from her distressing condition, which can be achieved by controlling the asthma with the very effective treatments now available.

Until last year, when another decline in Sara's health demanded that I should return to live in Britain with my two children, while my husband remained working abroad, I had not had the opportunity to cast around to try to find out more about the extent of this disease and its effects, so absorbed was I in Sara's condition. After some time in England, despite excellent treatment of her illness by a vigorous team of doctors at the Leeds General Infirmary, I felt certain that somewhere there must be even more information available. So it was that I picked up the telephone and asked a most sympathetic gentleman from Directory Enquiries to try to locate an Asthma Society for me. He succeeded in record time, and directed my attention to the Asthma Society and Friends of the Asthma Research Council in London. I wrote to them immediately. I have been overwhelmed by their response, and now realise that much is being done in the struggle to combat this distressing condition, and that much still remains to be done in drawing the attention not only of the general public, but also of some of the medical profession, to the suffering which can be caused by this 'Cinderella' of illnesses.

The book which follows is not an attempt to construct a text or reference book on the subject of asthma; it is rather a direct result of my diary about Sara, combined with my own frustrations when I have scoured libraries and bookshops alike, trying in vain to find a book illustrating the 'layperson's' viewpoint and experience of asthma, to enable me to compare Sara's condition with that of her fellow asthmatics. I should also like to think that I can help other people to avoid some of the mistakes which I have made, and to assure you that searching the world for a 'magic cure' is a pointless endeavour. The most excellent treatment may very well be available on your own doorstep.

I offer Sara's story to her fellow sufferers and their relatives, in the sincere hope that it will be both interesting and supportive.

# PART I

## *SARA'S STORY*

# Chapter One

'Help me, Mummy, I can't breathe,' a small child gasps desperately, and you stand there foolishly, swamped with the knowledge of your own inadequacy. Doctors and nurses move swiftly about their various tasks. What are they doing? How critical is the situation? You cannot stop them now to ask. A child is fighting for her life. You, the one person whom she has always relied upon for comfort and for the solutions to life's myriad small problems, are suddenly rendered impotent, useless.

These were the feelings, somewhat inadequately expressed, of both my husband and myself, when, in April 1984, Sara, our then four-year-old daughter, was admitted as an emergency case to a large but somewhat spartanly equipped hospital on a small Mediterranean island. This particular asthma attack escalated in severity to one which eventually required her urgent admission to an intensive care unit—but more of that later.

Our story may at times seem incredible, and even a little melodramatic, but I have long since accepted the fact that the simple truth is very often more fantastic than fiction.

*       *       *

Sara's life began at one o'clock in the morning on 6th May, 1979. She was born in the homely surroundings of a nursing home, which was run by nuns on the Mediterranean island where we lived. Her parents, Steve and myself, were both highly successful, very much in love, and as yet largely untouched by any of life's problems. Our first meeting fulfils all the requirements of a romantic novel. I was a professional singer, having studied for a number of years at the Royal Northern College of Music before joining the D'Oyly Carte Opera Company. I then veered away towards the lighter side of 'the business', working on Children's Television and finally travelling extensively with my own cabaret act. It was during a working holiday abroad that I met Steve; he was running a large manufacturing company on the island. Within a week of meeting we were engaged, three months later married and, in a little under a year, Sara was born. Our doctor was enraptured by his first sight of Sara, and declared her to be the most beautiful baby he had ever delivered. This being my first child, I had expected to find my new-born baby florid and wrinkled like a rosy prune; instead I was handed a perfectly lovely little dark-haired doll.

I was utterly relieved to find her apparently perfect, and myself relatively unscathed, as my time in the nursing home had been more than a little unnerving, to say the least. To explain what I mean, it is necessary to spare a moment to enlighten the reader about various matters regarding modes of behaviour possibly peculiar to the Mediterranean temperament—at least where the process of birth is concerned. Rather than the solitary, pacing figure of the father-to-be, whom we have come to expect at such times, every corridor, window-ledge and staircase of my nursing home was peopled by the extended families, not to mention friends, of the expectant mothers. It was rather like a mass gathering of faithful supporters' clubs, set in for the duration of their party's labour, with gossip, sandwiches and bottles of beer. Brief silences engulf the boisterous assembly as the air is rent spasmodically with blood-curdling shrieks issuing from the mothers-to-be. I have it on good authority that the louder the screams, the greater will be the material reward for enduring this 'punishment'. I can only suppose that the day following Sara's birth must have been a 'boom time' for the local jewellers, as I produced her during a particularly noisy night! I maintained my 'stiff upper lip', with the aid of a cup of tea and a few choice expletives, while I wondered where I was going wrong with my breathing exercises.

We brought Sara home to an imposing sandstone villa, complete with large swimming pool, countless rooms and five bathrooms. This may all sound most impressive, but I think I should point out before I go any further that there was one thing missing . . . water! This would have been extremely useful, but is unfortunately at a premium in May, when the boreholes are running dry and the desalination plant breaks down.

Nothing daunted, we set about the task of caring for our new-born baby, with our trusty 'Mothercare' book opened at the appropriate page for bathtime, nappy folding and other essential activities. I should explain that neither Steve nor myself had the least experience with small babies. Our maid, Jane, who was about forty at this time, must have been one of the few unmarried women on the island who was not a nun. She shared our bafflement at the best way of coping with the ever increasing demands of the small intruder, who had turned our previously efficiently run household upside down. I had not had a chance to 'practise' with Sara in the nursing home, as my room had been rather like Piccadilly Circus, with constant parades of Steve's business associates, offering their congratulations and ever larger bouquets. I drew a complete blank with breastfeeding, too. The lack of privacy in the nursing home did not help, and the nuns, although immensely kind, obviously thought that this sort of thing was out of their province, and that babies were far better served by a nice sterile bottle in the nursery. Despite all this, babies are resilient little things and Sara managed to survive my clumsy ministrations. Revelling in our unaccountable success, fourteen months later we produced James.

Two happy, trouble-free years with our babies then passed, in our affluent cocoon. Then, like the proverbial people who have much but are never satisfied, the time came when we both wanted to spread our wings and escape what we saw as the confining limitations of life on a small island. So in 1981 we sold our house and made plans to come home to England for good. Looking back now, those first years seem like a magical time which never really happened, for when we tried to recreate that trouble-free life for ourselves a few years later, it proved to be just an unattainable illusion.

Steve's father and stepmother lived on the same island. They had both been extremely upset by the news of our decision to leave, although it is fair to say that they had had a hard time accepting my sudden and unexpected arrival into their family. Steve had always been such an intrinsic part of their lives; until I appeared, like a bolt out of the blue—a 'cabaret singer' who had not only become Steve's wife, but almost before they had had time to come to terms with that, the mother of two of their grandchildren. Small wonder they did not know what to make of it.

Whatever their feelings may have been at the time, they contained them with admirable restraint and threw a most memorable party in the lush, poolside gardens of their beautiful home to mark our departure. It was a glorious and carefree afternoon. Once the more serious business of farewells was concluded, we abandoned ourselves with ever-increasing fervour to dancing wild tarantellas with some irrepressible Italian friends who were holidaying with us at the time, and finally sang our way mercilessly through most of the better known Italian operas.

The following day found us, not surprisingly, somewhat subdued. Harsh reality follows hard on the heels of an early morning stumble through the bottles and ash debris of the 'night before'. Sara and James, just twenty-three months and nine months respectively, were still far too young to appreciate that they were leaving their sunny island home for good. Sara was infused with excitement at the thought of our forthcoming trip, especially the first part which was to take us to the mainland on the large ferry-boat she had seen in the harbour. Steve and I had decided to take our time going home, in order to see as much of Europe as possible, so we planned to drive rather than fly. Even now, though I realise it is totally illogical, I wonder whether Sara might never have encountered whatever it was that 'triggered off' her asthma, if we had flown straight home to England.

# Chapter Two

The ferry docked in Naples, and we went on from there to Rome by car. In Rome we were to meet up once again with our Italian friends. James and Sara sat happily in their matching car seats, and we considered ourselves to be very well organised, and quite definitely prepared for any eventuality. We had stuffed the car with every imaginable item of baby care equipment. Of course, neither child had suffered a day's illness before this time, so we had good reason to feel confident.

The first part of the trip exceeded our expectations. At the very last minute, Sara obliged us by deciding that nappies, night-time or otherwise, were now superfluous where she was concerned. A propitious start!

Rome was fabulous. Our Roman friends lavished hospitality upon us. We visited so many fascinating places which we might have missed as unaccompanied tourists. We ate in a multitude of different cafés and restaurants, both grand and casual. The children revelled in the chic ice-cream parlours where it is only possible to guzzle the disqustingly sweet icy confections with the aid of a glass of iced water or an espresso coffee.

Italians love children and, rather refreshingly, expect them to behave exactly as children and not as miniature adults. Our friends were no exception, and accordingly egged Sara on to all sorts of exciting new activities. With an elegant shrug they handed her a hose-pipe, and let her loose with it in their rambling garden, while we sat cool, not too collected, and extremely wet, as she attempted to master the art of directing the powerful stream of water. Next they took us on an exhausting tour of what must have been every children's boutique in Rome. James, being so young, was a fairly cool observer of all the carry-on, but Sara caught on fast. Hardly were we through the door of the latest emporium, before she ripped off her clothes with newly acquired Italian abandon and stood looking appealingly at row upon row of tastefully displayed dresses. It was hard to say no; we had had so little choice on our tiny island home. We were all so incredibly happy, the children must have thought it was Christmas every day. After initial attempts to fend off the effusive attention lavished upon Sara and James by complete strangers, Steve and I became passive observers, allowing Italian enthusiasm full rein. James, very blond, with large, serious blue eyes, would recline nonchalantly in his pushchair, calmly accepting their plaudits, while my vivacious daughter, with her wavy, dark hair and mischievous green eyes, soon become adept at 'playing to the gallery'.

We were taken aback to find that our friends' home had some rather unusual features. It was one of a number of large houses, located just outside the city, and contained within a fortified park. Armed guards and dogs patrolled constantly. Perhaps not such a good idea after all, we thought, somewhat sobered, to be rich and Roman.

On our last day in Rome we all went up into the hills above the city, where we enjoyed a riotous meal in surroundings which could only be Italian—a huge barn of a place, rafters reverberating to the crash of plates and upraised voices. Children scampered unhindered between the tables, families greeted one another across the platters of steaming food on the well-scrubbed tables. All had brought their own supply of home-made wine, which tasted misleadingly like blackcurrant juice yet packed a punch like dynamite! I do not think we have ever enjoyed ourselves more, and not surprisingly, as there was not a single reason why we should have a care in the world. Just before we left this happy place, we rashly purchased double our quota of duty-free wine and proceeded enthusiastically on to Venice.

The nightmare began there in Venice, in the uncompromisingly theatrical setting of animated Canalettos. Our senses reeled before the thought-provoking contradictions which were immediately self-evident in this beautiful yet mouldering city. Beauty, decay, pigeons and smells. A place I never want to return to, because there Sara's suffering began and our family's comfortable, care-free existence came to an abrupt halt.

We had spent the disappointingly overcast day as model tourists. A trip to the Murano glass factory, where the magnificently ornate chandeliers and delicate rainbow-hued Venetian glass ornaments are produced. We visited St Mark's square and sat watching the clouds of pigeons billow and stream above the towering relics of antiquity, before moving on to yet another of the fascinating museums, crumbling treasure-houses which lie waiting to be discovered in the narrow alleyways that flank the sour, stagnating water of the canals. And then, of course, a trip by gondola. It seems strangely prophetic now to examine our collection of snapshots and discover one of Sara sitting on my knee in the boat, already looking 'peaky', and the quaint road sign (no doubt the reason why Steve in his innocence took the shot), adapted for use over the canals, which appears suspended immediately over Sara's head in the picture, proclaiming 'Hospital'.

Noting Sara's ever-increasing lethargy, we decided that she must be overtired, and so we returned to the hotel and put her to bed for a rest. There was no real reason for us to be concerned, or so we thought. We had all had a hectic couple of weeks and the children were bound to be tired.

Sara fell asleep immediately and slept on and on, well into the evening. Steve and I showered and changed ready to go downstairs for our evening meal. We usually ate early with the children, before putting James to bed for the night. Still Sara slept; and so heavily that at last we began to feel a little uneasy. It was unnatural for Sara to be so still. She was sleeping as if she was drugged. Normally she was a light sleeper, being such a lively, curious child, and so constantly worried she might 'miss out' on something.

Sara did not seem to have a temperature, or show any other worrying symptoms, so I persuaded Steve to go down and have his meal, while I fed James in the room and kept an eye on Sara. By the time Steve returned, Sara had become restless, although she did not seem to be fully awake. Her breathing was a little fast and chesty, nothing terribly dramatic yet, but we were so shocked at any sign of illness in a child who had always been so completely healthy, that we decided to call a doctor straight away. Athough Steve speaks fluent Italian, he was unable to satisfy himself that the hotel's receptionist would summon a doctor immediately. The man assured Steve that yes, yes, he would call, but we were not convinced. It was growing quite late now; all the local surgeries were closed, and it would mean calling a doctor out from his home. Steve returned to the room and we sat together watching Sara anxiously. There was no improvement, and the doctor still had not come. Steve returned to the receptionist after a few minutes and repeated his request for a doctor. Apparently there followed much shrugging of shoulders and rolling of eyes, as the man maintained more stubbornly that the lateness of the hour now made it difficult, if not impossible, to find a doctor. He continued with this singularly unhelpful attitude until Steve produced a Lire note of sufficiently enticing value, whereupon he suddenly became the very model of efficiency. Like a rabbit out of a conjurer's hat a doctor's telephone number came to mind, and he dialled the number with a flourish. Unfortunately, I am inclined to think now, with the wisdom of hindsight, that he must have selected the most unreliable doctor he could think of, in the hope of further financial inducement.

After a long, increasingly worrying wait, an elderly doctor arrived. Whether his rolling gait was the result of an unusually rough ride on the canal, or of an excess of alcohol, which seems the more likely explanation, we shall never know. He gave Sara the most cursory examination and seemed disgruntled at having been called out. Sara was still restless, and breathing even more heavily. We recognise now that she must have been wheezing for some time, something a one-eyed Tibetan tribesman in his first year at medical school should have realised; but we did not and, more importantly, neither did the doctor. Sara's face was extremely flushed, yet she did not feel hot at all. The 'doctor' produced a bottle of antibiotic, charged us the equivalent of fifty pounds, and made a hasty if unsteady exit.

Events moved with terrifying speed as Sara's condition began to deteriorate rapidly. By now, she was grabbing frantically at the neck of her pyjamas, whose slight pressure was sufficient to cause her extreme discomfort. Her breathing was shallow and rapid and her face was livid, although her lips were tinged with blue. Both Steve and I realised that there was no more time to lose; we must do something and fast! Neither of us had ever encountered a situation like it before. We knew Sara needed help right away, no matter the time and whatever the cost. I raised her up on pillows and began to cut away the top of her pyjamas with a pair of nail scissors; she was too distressed by her inability to breathe for us to cover her mouth even for an instant by trying to pull the top over her head. Steve grabbed up all the loose money we had available and dashed frantically downstairs again in a fury, determined to motivate the sullen receptionist into action, whatever it took. It was the most appalling situation: stuck in a hotel room in a strange country, where I did not even speak the language; a useless receptionist downstairs; baby James asleep in his cot; and Sara, gripped by some frightful illness which we could not even begin to understand. Surely there must be a doctor somewhere who could help us. Thankfully, Steve's desperation must have communicated itself to the receptionist. He agreed to call another doctor who arrived within minutes and, taking one look at Sara, did not hesitate. He called an ambulance immediately and, despite our insistence to the contrary, he refused all payment.

We had decided that Steve must stay in the hotel with James who, with a sleeping baby's supreme indifference, had slept through the whole affair. I hardly know what I expected to find as I followed the doctor down the stairs, carrying Sara wrapped in a blanket. Had I been thinking clearly, I would not have been so surprised to board a fast motor launch, which was of course an ambulance Venetian style. An attendant helped us into the boat. I sat in the cabin and the doctor laid Sara on my knee. The two men had a brief discussion in Italian, and then, to my intense dismay, the doctor bowed politely, said goodbye to me and left. I had thought that he would accompany us to the hospital, and it was far too late to wish that my Italian-speaking husband could take my place. I think it is a pretty fair, if harsh, assessment to say that since meeting Steve up until this moment, I had not made a decision, taken a stand or scrubbed a floor—all that was about to change.

The ambulance attendant, who had seated himself on a bench opposite me, did not speak any English, and as I was equally ignorant of Italian, we had to content ourselves with exchanging understanding looks as we glanced at each other across the dimly lit cabin. At last the boat began to pull away from the hotel's landing stage. With a great roar, the throttles opened, the motor ambulance seemed to lift out of the water, and then a great surge of power propelled us away down the narrow canal at hair-raising speed. Soon we reached the open lagoon, and I willed the boat to go even faster, if possible, as I clung to Sara and wished her well again with every fibre of my being.

We soon arrived at the hospital. It was obvious that we were expected as a nurse stood waiting on the quayside, and Sara was whisked out of my arms and carried quickly out of sight into the building. I tried to follow but was stopped at the porter's lodge. I was desperate to reach Sara, but they would not let me go to her. Finally they made me understand that I must produce my passport; fortunately I had remembered to bring it with me. I handed it over and received a largely incomprehensible, detailed form in return. It was more important to be with Sara. I thrust the form back at the man and begged to be allowed to go to her. The porter seemed to find my protestations amusing, as he turned to chat with his companion and calmly handed the form back to me. I began to shout and, to put it as politely as possible, he gestured most insistently to the effect that I could not proceed another foot until I did as he asked. My loathing of bureaucracy must surely emanate from this moment. A patient could be breathing his last, but there would surely be an appropriate form for the attendant relative to fill in. My sum knowledge of the Italian language is unfortunately restricted to the pronunciation of same for the purposes of singing. We British are notoriously dismissive of those who cannot speak our own language, and it was quite a rôle reversal to find myself in the part of the uncomprehending foreigner, who both feels and is assumed to be, an idiot. Complication followed misunderstanding as I blundered through the paperwork necessary for Sara's admission.

Finally, sweating and seething with frustration, I managed to complete the form to the man's satisfaction, and was allowed to enter the hospital. I joined Sara in a small cubicle where she was being examined by a doctor, and I felt even worse now, hovering on the sidelines, not understanding a single word that was being said about her. It was by now the middle of the night and the hospital had only a skeleton staff on duty, none of whom spoke English. Sara was either asleep or unconscious, I had to idea which; she lay completely still, but her breathing was rapid and noisy. She was moved into a small side room, and a nurse came and held her on her knee while she gave her some medication, which Sara inhaled through a mask. She was completely limp as she lay across the nurse's lap, except for the convulsive bellows-motion of her tiny chest.

The nurse, who had taken my place, helping Sara when I could do nothing, was very kind. She rocked Sara gently as if she was holding her own small child, and her eyes told me that she knew and understood my fears, even though she was unable to speak to me.

I know now that Sara could have died in Venice as a result of this acute attack remaining untreated for so long. Death from asthma is rare, but those who suffer from chronic asthma are most at risk. Sadly, it was to be some time before we were told that Sara was asthmatic, let alone that her condition was extremely serious. There always has to be the first experience, the one you do not understand or recognise for what it is; this was just the case for us in Venice. It is imperative to be able to decide when an attack is becoming dangerous, as most deaths occur in the home, rather than in hospital. This is usually because the severity of the attack has not been appreciated, and so the necessary treatment has not been started. I did not discover for some time that even the intensity of the wheeze can be misleading, as sometimes a further deterioration in the child's condition can lead to an almost silent chest. Help is needed urgently if the child appears blue (cyanosed) in any way, is becoming obviously exhausted by her condition, or is no longer fully conscious. Bitter experience with Sara has taught me to check her fingernails and the area around her mouth for the most obvious signs that she has a blue tinge, although I must emphasise that my vigilance, subsequent to our experience in Venice, has been required beside a hospital bedside.

Once Sara's condition became so obvious that she was actually diagnosed asthmatic, and I knew exactly what I was dealing with, there was no way that I would wait until any of the above-mentioned symptoms had become apparent before I took her to the nearest casualty department. All the signs I mention above are *late* signs, *denoting a critical condition.* I would now take Sara into hospital immediately, should she fail to respond to her nebulised solution of the popular bronchodilator, Ventolin, within the ten minutes or so it takes her to inhale the drug. I shall explain this treatment in Part II of the book; it is one which I administer at the first sign of a wheeze. If she showed any of the symptoms of cyanosis, I would not try anything myself at home; I would take her straight to hospital. Of Sara's innumerable hospital admissions, many of which have been severe, some have been false alarms. In Britain I have never been made to feel that I was 'crying wolf'. Doctors would far rather treat children in the earliest stages of an attack and send them home, than cope with the chronic results of a parent waiting too long for fear of being a nuisance.

It has been said to me recently that, although a very mild asthmatic condition may remain unrecognised as such for some time, an acute asthma attack could never be mistaken —unless, of course, you were rather 'dumb'. Perhaps I was unusually slow in identifying Sara's illness but, coming from a family which had been fortunate in never encountering a serious illness, and never having known anyone asthmatic or witnessed an asthmatic attack, I assumed that Sara was suffering from an acute viral infection which she had picked up on our travels. I do not have the benefit of intensive medical training, which would have equipped me with the acute perception necessary to recognise immediately the relevant symptoms, and, unfortunately, the insurmountable language barrier prevented the doctors in Venice from explaining to me the nature of Sara's illness.

When she had completed the treatment prescribed for her during that long night in Venice, Sara was put into a hospital bed and an oxygen tent was erected around her. I was more frightened still, as this in itself seemed to denote a much more serious condition than I had at first assumed. Oxygen tents to the medical profession are usual and commonplace objects; to the layperson they are emotive paraphernalia which are seldom, if ever, encountered. I sat on a chair at Sara's side throughout the night, and watched anxiously for any signs of improvement. Gradually her breathing returned to normal, her colour returned, she regained consciousness and recognised me. By the early hours of the morning she was full of life, but absolutely terrified by the oxygen tent. She kept trying to get out of bed and became very distraught, crying out repeatedly for Daddy and Jamie . . . 'Where's this? Where's this?' she kept asking frantically. She fought me off as I tried to keep her in the bed. 'Why Mummy? Why?'—I am quite sure I did not come up with a satisfactory explanation. Unable to calm her, I crept under the tent and lay down beside her, holding her close, but the nurses caught me and hauled me out again. I still had no idea what was wrong with her or what was right or wrong to do; I was just following my instincts and trying to comfort her as much as possible.

In the morning a doctor arrived to examine Sara. Her knowledge of English was minimal but sufficient to be able to explain to me that Sara was no longer 'in danger'. I can still quite clearly remember my feelings of bewilderment. Sara, in danger? In danger of what? . . . Dying . . .? And now the same doctor was calmly telling me that Sara would be discharged in two days' time! It was all totally incomprehensible.

In that remarkable manner which seems peculiar to children, Sara bounced back to health in record time. I stayed with her in the hospital, and we waved at Daddy and James through the window when they came to visit us. I should explain that there was a measles epidemic in Venice at the time; consequently no visitors were allowed inside the hospital. Sara adapted to her brief stay with amazing speed and was soon able to hold mini-conversations with the staff—very humbling for myself!

On the third day she was discharged. I was handed a discharge note in a sealed envelope, which I naturally ripped open as soon as we reached the hotel. To our disappointment, it only showed proof of her admission to hospital, with the relevant dates. No information regarding a diagnosis of her illness was shown.

# Chapter Three

I flew straight back to England with the children, leaving Steve behind in Venice to follow on with the car and all our luggage. I had already decided that my best plan would be to stay with my mother in Yorkshire for the time being, and to get Sara examined as quickly as possible while we waited for Steve to arrive. After a night's sleep I left James with my mother and took Sara to see the local GP.

I gave the doctor a detailed account of what I understood about Sara's illness in Venice, naturally mentioning both the time she had spent in an oxygen tent, and also the fact that some medications had been administered through a mask—and that the latter had seemed to assist her breathing quite considerably. The doctor gave Sara a thorough examination and pronounced her fit. As his thoughts echoed my own, it seemed quite reasonable to hear him suggest the possibility that she had picked up a virus infection on our travels. I am not by nature a cynical person, but now I wonder what we would all do without that all-encompassing diagnosis, 'the virus infection'.

Possibly the doctor suspected that Sara had suffered an asthma attack, but asthma is not easy to diagnose, and must certainly be less so when all you have to go on is a second-hand account of what happened—and that from an unqualified observer. He went on to assure me that Sara was now in perfect health; the illness in Venice was almost certainly an isolated incident, requiring no further treatment or investigation. In fairness to the doctor, I have to say that even now, when Sara is a known asthmatic, between her attacks she appears to be an absolutely normal, healthy little girl. I left the surgery feeling immensely relieved, certain that the whole episode had simply been a ghastly blot on our otherwise trouble-free lives. How wrong can one be?

Our family's luck had taken a definite turn for the worse. Steve had decided, in his concern to be with myself and the children, to drive literally without stopping from Venice to Yorkshire. He drove through the worst excesses of traffic in Europe on what was now Easter Sunday, caught the last ferry from Calais, and arrived in Dover both exhausted and extremely impatient to be with us and to know what the doctor had had to say about Sara. He also brought with him all our essential luggage, which I had left behind in my eagerness to get home. Because of this combination of exceptional factors, his tiredness rendered him vulnerable to certain suggestions made by customs officials in Dover, supposedly to cut through a lot of the 'red tape' which surrounds the importation of cars into this country. Steve was only too willing to comply with anything which would ensure his speedy departure from Dover, and regrettably made the mistake of thinking that the suggestions had been made out of sympathy for his story about Sara, which he had told the officials in the hope that they would speed things up for him. A costly 'misunderstanding' followed, which caused our car to be seized—and I might add that our wine disappeared at the same time, although no mention of wine, excess or otherwise, was made at the time. An ironic footnote to Steve's unfortunate experience was that the very next day there was a strike by customs officers, and all the posts at Dover were unmanned.

There now followed a truly terrible time; a part of our lives which, if I could, I would happily erase. Our total lack of understanding of Sara's condition, coupled with our complete trust in the diagnoses of several doctors over the ensuing months, led to a period of intolerable strain for Steve and myself, plus, more importantly, a lot of unnecessary distress for Sara.

We had decided to settle in London, and bought a house in a typical, leafy suburb. The children seemed to adjust happily enough to their new home, except for one disturbing thing: Sara, could not, or would not, as we wrongly thought at the time, sleep at all. Every single night she coughed continuously. The deterioration was swift and insidious. An occasional sleepless night progressed rapidly to weeks and then months of sleepless nights. I thought I would go mad; my body felt like a concrete overcoat during the day and, at night, Steve and I would crawl into bed always hoping that this night would be different. Sometimes we would manage to doze for a few hours, until the all-too inevitable sound of Sara's nerve-racking cough woke us yet again. The strain of waiting, stranded somewhere between sleep and consciousness, night after night, became desperate. I took Sara repeatedly to our local doctor's surgery. The bewildering fact was that she appeared to be perfectly well during the day and, unlike us, practically unaffected by the lack of sleep. The doctor would examine this amazingly healthy-looking child, listen carefully to her chest and then inform me, with growing impatience, that there was nothing wrong with her. He obviously thought there was something wrong with me! After many visits the doctor must have been at his wits' end, too, for finally he made the suggestion which, far from reassuring us, only aggravated our concern. He asserted that as Sara was obviously in perfect health, we were encountering an emotional problem; Sara was jealous of Mummy and Daddy sleeping together. Although the doctor assured us that some little girls have this problem, I can certainly say that this possibility had never crossed my mind.

Our doctor maintained that some children will stop at

nothing to capture their parents' full attention, even to the extent of keeping them awake all night. He warmed to his theme and said that Sara was using her cough as a ploy to make me leave Steve and stay with her. Well, of course I comforted Sara during these attacks, sometimes in her bed and sometimes in ours. She is a very warm and loving little girl and, like all children, responds well to affection; she tried so hard to subdue the appalling coughing fits when we soothed her with a cuddle. I did not give up with the doctor, but persisted in stressing on each visit that the night-time cough was extremely upsetting for Sara, and showed no sign of abating; surely something could be done. Each time I was assured, with studied politeness, that there was nothing at all to worry about, before being ushered out of the surgery.

If only once, during the dreadful months which followed, the doctor had put the easy options of 'virus infection' and 'emotional disturbance' out of his mind, and given some real thought to Sara's condition, he must surely have considered the possibility that she was an asthmatic child. If only I had known, I would have been able to research the illness and understand, as I do now, that asthma is often at its worst during the night, especially in children under five years old. How angry I feel now, to know that it is almost always possible to prevent continuous night-time coughing; indeed this is now the case with Sara. As it was, time passed, Steve and I remained unable to have a full night's sleep, and the atmosphere in our home began to deteriorate. It was like living on a knife-edge; patience was at a premium, and Steve and I spent all our time snapping and shouting at each other, while staring balefully at poor little Sara, the object of our discomfort. We found it impossible to come to terms with the fact that this was some sort of emotional phase which she would eventually 'grow out of'. I cannot say that it was just the lack of sleep; having had two babies, we, like all other parents, had suffered our share of interrupted nights. It was more the fact that we had been told quite clearly that there was no good reason for these interrupted nights, which finally wore us down. I can still recall with utter horror the night when, absolutely at the end of my tether, I stormed into Sara's room and began shaking her as I screamed and cried, begging her to please let us have some sleep.

Our chronic tiredness and sense of frustration had created a vicious circle which made us progressively less sympathetic to Sara's condition. To any parents who are presently experiencing this nightmare for themselves, I urge you to go along to your local hospital, explain the situation and see if your child can be admitted for a few nights while you have a rest. You may find that the cough recurs, despite proper medication for asthma. This is possibly because the child's condition is temporarily exacerbated by a cold, or stress.

It is so easy for me to look back now and know, with absolute certainty, that long before we reached this stage I should have insisted that the GP refer Sara to a chest consultant—and if he refused to do so, take her to the nearest hospital myself. I was actually beginning to feel that the doctor's obvious opinion of me as a 'neurotic mother', might contain an element of truth; after all, Sara did look marvellously well during the day, and it did seem that her coughing began every night, soon after Steve and I went to bed. Being befuddled with tiredness, I lacked the energy required to act more decisively in getting to the bottom of the problem.

It seems hardly possible now, but things got worse—the racking cough combined with a sudden 'rush' of catarrh onto her chest. This was sometimes so severe that Sara was violently sick. Naturally this caused her extreme distress and we were obliged, on a number of occasions, to call out the doctor in the middle of the night. He always examined Sara carefully, and his advice was to boil a kettle of water in her room and prop her up on pillows. As for his diagnosis, it was 'childish wheezing'—something which, according to him, occurs in many children, is nothing to worry about and, once again, she would soon 'grow out of it'. And, yes, we *had* told him all about the frightening experience in Venice. Steve and I could not believe that was all; we were extremely worried and suggested to the doctor that it must surely be a good idea for Sara to visit a chest specialist—and would he please refer us to one. The doctor told us that we were wasting our time as there was really nothing more to add to the information which he had already given us; moreover, we would also be wasting the specialist's time. He pointed to Sara's throat and also her ribcage. He said that we need only be concerned if we could see the flesh being sucked in and out rapidly in an involuntary spasmodic movement, coupled with a blue tinge around her mouth. Even in our ignorance, this all sounded rather like sitting around, foolishly waiting for a condition to deteriorate from bad to chronic, before taking any action. Now I find it quite incredible and would beseech you to move immediately in the direction of your nearest hospital's Casualty Department, long before any such deterioration occurs.

Childish wheezing, sometimes referred to as wheezy bronchitis, is just another form of asthma. This was never made clear to me in the early days of Sara's illness—and that, above all, is why I failed to understand her condition.

By far the commonest cause of wheezing over a prolonged period is an infection of the nose and possibly the throat. This is particularly so in the early years of life, when the inflammation which accompanies the infection is likely to cause the airway muscles to contract, and the lining to swell and weep. Unfortunately for Sara, it was to be a matter of years rather than weeks before any doctor referred to her as 'asthmatic', thus enabling me, at last, to read more about the disease and understand exactly what we were dealing with. In all the time I wasted, labouring under the misconception that wheezy bronchitis or childish wheezing was something you must endure or, at worst, a condition you just 'took a pill for' and it would obligingly go away, never once did asthma occur to me.

In order to clarify the point about wheezy bronchitis, Hugh Faulkner, Director of the Asthma Society and Friends of the Asthma Research Council, kindly put me in touch with two experts in this field of medicine, Dr Frankland and Professor A.D. Milner who is Professor of Paediatric Respiratory Medicine at University Hospital, Nottingham. Professor Milner states:

> The term 'wheezy bronchitis' is often used to describe the wheezing which comes on within one or two days of the onset of a cold. It occurs most commonly in the first three years of life. *This is just a form of asthma* and responds to treatment in exactly the same way as asthma brought on by allergy. Some doctors are reluctant to use the word asthma as they feel they will frighten and upset the child's parents. I think it preferable to spend time explaining the nature of asthma, how it will almost always respond to treatment and the excellent long-term outlook for many.

If only we had encountered Professor Milner five years ago; thank goodness for his down to earth approach. Like him, I fail to see the point in lulling parents into a false sense of security, thus exposing the asthmatic child to unnecessary suffering—and even risk to her life. In order to react swiftly and responsibly to a situation, parents must first understand fully the nature of the illness.

Dr Frankland's comments on the subject serve to emphasise Sara's doctors' incredible oversight. He says:

The point about 'childish wheezing' is that in one group of children, the wheezing occurs only with infective episodes, and for this reason is nearly always called bronchitis. The outlook in this group is generally very good. Not so in the child where there is a family history of allergy, the complaint has been preceded by eczema and the child is in the allergic group. It is just in this group that the wheezing, although triggered to begin with by infection, may have a definite spasmodic element to it and should be called asthma. It is very difficult to diagnose asthma under the age of one. We must remember that many so-called 'wheezy bronchitics' are *not* bronchitics at all, but are asthmatics. It is for this reason that *any* wheezing in a child should be investigated, or at least thought of as asthmatic, and the causes are not necessarily due to infection. The wheezing has nothing to do with 'immature airways'. Increased secretions, swelling of the lining and spasm —any of these three can cause wheezing at any age, young or old.

I am quite sure that by now the reader will find it strange that we were still totally oblivious to the true nature of Sara's illness. Indeed, I find it hard myself to accept today that the possibility that Sara might be asthmatic had still not occurred to either of us. The reason is simple: I was old-fashioned enough to believe that the doctor knows best, which he should, having had many years of intensive training. If I had been asked for my definition of an asthmatic at this time, I should probably have said that an asthmatic was someone extremely frail, semi-invalid, who found constant difficulty in breathing, even to the extent of being frequently confined to bed with acute breathing problems. A rather vague notion, I am afraid, and certainly not someone who resembled my extremely robust, sturdy little girl in the least. The one similarity in Sara's case to my idea of an asthmatic was her 'bad chest', and this condition had been dismissed reassuringly by several doctors as the result of frequent virus infections.

Sara's third birthday was approaching rapidly and we planned a party which was to be held in our garden for Sara, James and all their friends. I had begun to realise that excitement of any kind seemed to aggravate her cough, and I was therefore careful to keep all the party preparations extremely low-key. The eagerly anticipated day drew closer, my parents arrived from Yorkshire and it became increasingly difficult to satisfy Sara's constant enquiries about the progress of plans for her party, and to keep her calm at the same time. One thing I have noticed about my daughter time and time again is that, although excitement aggravates her condition, she seems to find a perverse satisfaction in 'winding herself up', rather like a little lemming dashing eagerly towards the inevitable precipice.

Sara's birthday dawned bright and sunny, but yes, you have guessed, Sara was by now confined to bed. She was flushed, lethargic, her breathing rapid and noisy—a condition which now, after so much more experience, I as a 'layperson' would have no difficulty in identifying as an asthmatic attack. Her party was cancelled and the doctor summoned. He prescribed an antibiotic, suggested that we should boil a kettle of water in her room, and thought it might also help if she were to inhale the steam from a bowl of hot water containing Friar's Balsam. All excellent suggestions for a 'bunged up' nose, no doubt—but for Sara? Yes, I am angry when I look back at this time. With the correct diagnosis and appropriate medication, my child could have avoided so much suffering from this constant, debilitating illness.

Thankfully, even without the benefit of appropriate medication, Sara made a gradual recovery from this attack and, after a few days in bed, returned to her usual bubbly self. A few discreet arrangements ensured that a completely 'surprise' birthday party could be held a week later, and Sara celebrated her third birthday with delight, her pleasure unspoiled by the return of her 'mystery' illness.

Without question, the numerous 'clues' to Sara's condition should have been glaring her doctor in the face. She was showing a fairly typical response by any asthmatic to an increase in stress—which in Sara's case was the result of her excited anticipation regarding the forthcoming birthday party. It would be wrong of me to suggest that excitement or anxiety precipitates asthma in a person who has never suffered from the disease before, but it is true to say that an existing condition may be aggravated by stress. Having said this, it is important that an asthmatic child is encouraged to lead as normal a life as possible; consequently, mollycoddling is *out*. Not so long ago I spoke to the parent of an asthmatic child, who told me that she never scolded her daughter in case the child became upset and had an attack; I am afraid that I do not subscribe to this approach. You cannot wrap a child in cotton-wool and kid yourself that you are doing her a favour; after all, she must face up to life sooner or later. Only recently Sara shrieked at my mother in aggrieved indignation, 'You can't tell me off, I'm asthmatic,' to which my mother responded calmly, 'So what? I'm diabetic. These things don't entitle us to any special privileges.' Obviously there are the rare cases of children who can actually bring on attacks when under pressure, and this is perhaps a signal that extra help is needed. It may even be necessary to call in a child specialist or seek advice at a child guidance clinic. It is out of the question for you to submit to emotional blackmail, as this will only make normal family life impossible, and impair your child's emotional development.

During the months following Sara's third birthday, the progressive deterioration in her health became more obvious. She still coughed during the night as usual, but now the bouts of so-called 'virus infections' occurred more frequently, so that she had no sooner recovered from one episode before she began to show signs of sickening with the next. The constant reassurances by our doctors in London were beginning to wear a little thin and we were more concerned than ever about Sara's continued ill-health. The slightest infection or excitement was sure to confine her to bed now, in what we both considered to be far too worrying a condition to be yet again dismissed lightly as 'childish wheezing', brought on by infection, or some sort of emotional irregularity. Paradoxically, Sara always appeared to be in the rudest of health during those rapidly decreasing periods between her attacks.

I simply could not understand what was happening and, more importantly, why the doctors could not do anything for Sara. At the same time, Steve's business interests were demanding more and more of his time, and he spent much of the time out of the country. We both agreed that I must have the support of my parents during his many absences; apart from assistance needed caring for Sara during her frequent illnesses, James was all too often being consigned to the sidelines. It was impossible to devote the amount of time which I knew he needed both to stimulate and reassure him, so we took the only option open to us and, in September 1982, sold our house in London, moving to Harewood in North Yorkshire, near to my parents' home.

The moment we were settled I sought out the doctor in our small village and told him all about Sara. This was our first major breakthrough. He did not dismiss me abruptly with yet another bottle of antibiotic, cough medicine, or any other variation on an ill-considered theme. He listened quietly and for quite some time, I remember, as I related every small detail which had contributed to our concern. He referred Sara immediately to a children's specialist in the area and, at long last, I felt that we were getting somewhere.

# Chapter Four

When the eagerly awaited day arrived, Sara was suffering, yet again, from one of her increasingly frequent 'bad chests'. The specialist questioned me closely about her and gave her a thorough external examination which, from his comments at the time, obviously did not give him much cause for concern. However, as he was naturally determined to get to the bottom of Sara's problem, he decided to send her for a chest X-ray.

Sara and I left his room coughing in concert. I had become so strung up simply thinking about the wonderful possibility that Sara would soon be well again, that I had developed a nervous cough which was completely beyond my control—much to the alarm of the technicians in the X-ray department, who were only expecting one small child with a cough. They told me later that they had all listened with amazement as we approached their room and had wondered what kind of small child could make such a terrible racket! Unfortunately, my desperate optimism was a little naïve; I should have known that things are rarely so simple.

Sara's X-ray showed that she was suffering from pneumonia. The specialist assured me that, however bad this might sound, in this instance he would be able to treat her illness in the comfortingly familiar surroundings of her own home. Even so, I was quite naturally extremely upset— from summary dismissal by our doctors in London, to this.

I could not help remembering how I had shouted at Sara in my frustration, months before, because I had been led to believe that her cough was the result of some sort of attention-grabbing emotional disorder. I still wonder what Sara's true condition may have been when I took her along, so very frequently, to the surgery in London, where she was only ever given a cursory external examination. My fears were further substantiated by something which happened much later, while Sara's condition (having been identified as asthma) was being closely monitored by an excellent team of doctors at Leeds General Infirmary. Despite an extensive programme of medications used to control her condition, she suffered, quite unexpectedly, from a recurrence of the unpleasant night-time cough, which we all had good reason to believe had disappeared for good. I took her straight in to Ward 56 in the Clarendon Wing of the Infirmary, where there is an 'open door' policy for Sara. A doctor examined her carefully and told me that her condition did not sound too serious. However, being fully aware of her past history, the doctor ordered a chest X-ray to be taken 'just as a precaution'. Despite this doctor's optimism, the results proved, yet again, that Sara was suffering from pneumonia, and she was admitted to the hospital immediately.

It had been explained to me that Sara's pneumonia, or pneumonitis, as it is more properly called, results from a mucus 'plug' forming in the lungs during an asthma attack. If infection also develops, she then has pneumonia. During the attack the air tubes in the lungs are narrowed, making breathing difficult. These irritated airways produce too much thick, sticky mucus which may form a 'plug', thus blocking off a section of the fine branches of the lungs. As there is no cross-branching in the lungs, the branches which lie beyond the 'plug' are completely starved of air, and so they collapse.

This collapse, in Sara's case, can be reversed by using

energetic physiotherapy, which literally helps to shake the 'plug' loose. This is achieved by a thrice-daily application of something half-way between a pat and a thump, to all the external areas over her lungs, while she is lying in a forward-tilting position, thus allowing the mucus to flow out of her lungs and eventually be coughed up. If she also has an infection, a course of antibiotics is usually necessary, too, to eliminate this.

'Pneumonia' and 'collapse' are extremely emotive words. At one time there was very good reason for this, as without the medicines available today, pneumonia could certainly strike down an apparently normally healthy person in the prime of life. Nowadays, it is an illness which usually responds quickly to treatment by antibiotics and so is no longer regarded as a necessarily life-threatening condition. Indeed, while the battle was still on to find a way to control Sara's asthma, she suffered from pneumonia with approximately the same frequency that most other children might catch a cold. If detected in the early stages, it was sometimes possible to treat her as an outpatient, applying physiotherapy on a regular basis, and taking a course of antibiotics.

With regard to the countless X-rays which Sara has had during the past five years, I have noticed a marked tendency by some doctors to refer to 'abnormal chest signs'. I am sure that this is meant to be a reassuring mode of expression for use before patients and relatives; I can only say that for me, these vague euphemisms conjured up all sorts of terrifying possibilities. I would like 'doctor-speak' to be abolished immediately, and ask, whenever possible, to be supplied with the true facts, clearly stated. When I badgered one young doctor to define 'abnormal', with regard to Sara's condition, he told me reluctantly that she actually had pneumonia. . . . but we don't use that word any more because it frightens people'. Well, in that instance, I was almost relieved to hear that Sara had a condition which I knew would respond well to treatment, rather than some irreversible and possibly fatal illness.

I experienced my first dose of 'doctor-speak' when the specialist, having scanned Sara's X-rays, remarked rather vaguely that there was a possibility she might be an 'allergic child'. Once again, no mention of asthma. My thoughts rattled away onto a branch line, which proved to be completely the wrong track. I am allergic, too,—to base metals and perfume. Providing my skin does not come into contact with them, I have no problem. Fantastic! I rejoiced—all we do now is find out what Sara is allergic to and remove it. What could be simpler?

We left the surgery in high spirits and I told Sara that she was going to be well all the time from now on; after all, it would not take me long to find out what she was allergic to. She was to take a course of antibiotics at home and, when she was a little better, attend the hospital as an outpatient for physiotherapy. Now the fun began. From the very beginning Sara hated her sessions with the physiotherapist. He was an extremely unsympathetic, well-muscled chap, whose brusque manner was probably better suited to dealing with reassembling the bodily machinery of rugby forwards, rather than caring for a tiny, three-year-old girl with pneumonia. He absolutely terrified Sara by ordering her to 'cough something up' after his vigorous sessions. Sara obviously imagined that something horrible would suddenly leap out of her throat if she tried too hard. Despite all our efforts to reassure her, she became progressively less co-operative. One thing I should dearly love to know—and this goes for some doctors, too,—whatever happened to the 'bedside manner'? Surely a little compassion is not too much to expect. After a couple of torture sessions, Sara decided, not unnaturally, that she would have nothing more to do with this man. She became completely hysterical if we even attempted to take her anywhere near him, and nothing I could say would convince her that there was no lurking demon existing deep down in the hidden recesses of her chest, only waiting for the golden opportunity to be 'coughed up'. After much patient counselling, I finally managed to persuade her that 'Mr Cough' was really something of a dimwit and could be spat out with relish. From then on we undertook the treatment ourselves at home. Sara responded marvellously to my energetic therapy, which we had turned into a game, and there were more laughs than tears as we worked together to 'evict' Mr Cough from his temporary lodgings.

After a week or so we returned to the specialist for further investigations. He continued to refer to Sara as an allergic child, and decided that she must now undergo a series of skin tests to try to identify what was causing her 'allergic reactions'. This procedure involved tiny drops of known allergens suspended in liquid being put on her arm, and then a scratch with a pin assured their absorption. Allergens are substances which cause an allergic reaction when they come into contact with the body of certain people, e.g., pollen, house dust, animal skin dust (dander), mould spores, certain foods, etc.

Sara bore the scratches bravely, as I explained to her carefully that we would soon see what was making her ill by the red bumps which would appear on her arm at any moment. The nurses must have thought I was mad, but no one disillusioned me! How I longed for some large, ugly red bumps to appear; these, I hoped, would identify the particular allergen(s) responsible for Sara's condition. I basked in my innocence, still imagining that I would then simply remove whatever it was that caused her sickness and all would be well. We were all to be disappointed—not a bump in sight. I did not know it then, but this result was all the more amazing because in fact more than 30 per cent of non-asthmatic children can have some positive skin tests.

The specialist seemed unconcerned with these rather

inconclusive results. He commented that skin tests are notoriously unreliable at the best of times, and have frequently been known to show positive results when a substance was already known to be harmless to the patient; or, indeed, negative results when a recognised 'trigger' was placed in contact with the patient. He also informed me blithely that it would be unusual for positive results to be obtained from these tests on such a young child. I was extremely irritated by this explanation, which I saw as a face-saving exercise. My feelings were that in skin tests are so unreliable and inconclusive, why inflict this unpleasant experience on Sara?

Still, out of all this came some real good. The specialist now mentioned asthma for the first time as the possible cause of Sara's distress. He explained to us that asthma is quite a common condition which affects the lungs, causing attacks of wheezing breathlessness and coughing, but that once it was possible to identify whatever might be 'triggering' Sara's attacks, her condition could be controlled. (I do not want to dampen all your hopes, but five years later it is still impossible to be sure exactly what causes Sara to have an asthma attack.) Although we were very upset, it was rather like the sun coming out; we had something positive to cling to at last. We rushed off eagerly, to carry out all the suggested precautions necessary for the maintenance of good health in an allergic asthmatic. Amongst the many, we covered Sara's mattress with a plastic envelope to protect her from the 'house dust mite' (see p. 125). This disgusting little creature is one of the commonest causes of allergic asthma—or, as one of the more humorous doctors I have met puts it, mite is right!

All Sara's soft toys were removed, as these can also harbour the dreaded mite. However, I must admit that I did let her keep one particularly precious bear, as he was washable. We replaced her carpet with easily washable vinyl floor covering and took away her feather duvet and pillows, replacing these with polyester bedding. Although the house dust mite is present in the cleanest home and virtually impossible to eliminate completely, I became obsessed with maintaining an immaculate standard of dust-free cleanliness in Sara's room at all times. Unfortunately for Sara, despite my most energetic efforts, in her case they proved to be a complete waste of time; she still coughed continuously, all night long.

Much was now expected of three-year-old Sara. She had begun to inhale a nebulised solution of Sodium Cromoglycate, commonly known as Intal, three times a day. This drug is a preventative treatment and must be taken regularly. Intal acts by making the walls of the airways less sensitive to irritants, and we administered it by using a nebuliser. This is a machine about the size of a portable radio, which forces compressed air through a flexible plastic tube, leading to a 'pipe'. Through this Sara was to draw and inhale the ensuing vapour—rather like an eastern hubble-bubble. Not surprisingly, it proved to be an almost impossible task for such a young child. Sometimes she had to sit for as long as forty minutes, while she struggled to master the art of sucking and inhaling; why the specialist had contrived such an awkward system for Sara, I have no idea. Later, we became thoroughly familiar with the flexible plastic face masks which are more commonly used—although we did not realise this at the time, and assumed that the method of treatment suggested by the specialist would be the most effective in Sara's case. The flexible face mask fits firmly over the nose and mouth area and the vaporised drug is pumped into it by the nebuliser machine; it does not require any active participation on the part of the patient. When another doctor, at a later stage, found Sara's 'hubble-bubble' rather perplexing and immediately suggested the use of the mask as a preferable alternative, we found that we could administer the same amount of solution in about five minutes.

Luckily for me, Sara has never objected to using a face mask, although I can imagine that this might be a problem with some very young children. The nebuliser is quite a noisy machine, which could be one factor that might frighten a small child. Perhaps you could leave it running with just some water in the container so that your child could have a look at it, see how it works, watch the mist puffing out and so become totally relaxed and familiar with the machine.

Children are unlikely to sit like little lambs for a full five minutes, unless there is something interesting to play quietly with, or listen to. A story, or even a television programme, would be a good idea; something to look forward to, so that the treatment becomes a secondary consideration. That should remove the fear, then, as the child begins to derive benefit from the treatment and is old enough to understand, she will welcome the treatment for its own sake. Older children might feel self-conscious about taking the drugs this way within sight of their friends, and it might be possible for your specialist to ensure that this sort of regular medication is taken night and morning, in the privacy of the child's own room.

Yet again we returned to the specialist, for although Sara's chest X-rays showed that the pneumonia had cleared from her lungs, she was still becoming ill far too frequently. The coughing continued without respite, and the days when she would be lively and completely untroubled by any 'bad chests', or extreme lethargy, grew fewer. She seemed to be spending almost all her time in bed, unable to attend the local kindergarten or play with her friends. The specialist now suggested the implementation of a stringent dietary procedure, in case Sara was reacting adversely to a certain food, or to the various additives which are present in almost all the foods we eat. I was to become increasingly aware of the amazing number of chemical additives which lace even the most mundane items found on the supermarket shelves. Sara's exclusion diet began with allowing her to eat those foods which are known to be 'safe' or inactive. We had great fun trying to interest our three-year-old in the respective merits of rice cereal in its various forms, lamb, carrots, honey and goat's milk. I devised all sorts of interesting concoctions, with, I might add, a varying degree of success. Gradually, month by month, we introduced certain groups of foods, until eventually Sara was eating normally again. Sadly for Sara, this did not seem to be the answer, either; her asthmatic condition remained constant throughout.

Despite our findings, or lack of them, I am still very wary about foods which are obviously loaded with colourings and chemicals, such as cola, orange squash, coloured cheese, etc. There are alternatives to these products and, although they do not seem to aggravate Sara's asthma, I am simply not keen on the idea of her regularly downing such vast quantities of unnecessary chemicals.

We had reached another dead end with Sara, because the exclusion diet had failed to prove anything conclusive about her condition. We were extremely conscientious regarding her treatment with the nebulised solution of Intal, and even though the specialist had now prescribed Alupent syrup in addition, for Sara to take whenever an attack threatened, nothing seemed to help. Alupent is a commonly used bronchodilator. In asthmatics, the air tubes in the lungs (bronchial tubes or bronchi) are narrowed, making breathing difficult. A bronchodilator is a substance which causes these narrowed tubes to open up, or dilate. Alupent syrup takes about 20 to 30 minutes to become effective, then it acts directly on the smooth muscle of the bronchial tube, causing it to lengthen and relax. I never found this syrup to be of much use for Sara, because it took too long to become effective, by which time her condition was too severe to receive sufficient benefit from this medicine alone. The syrup is, however, very useful in a child who only suffers from occasional, mild attacks.

The most effective way to administer a bronchodilator for the treatment of an asthma attack is to use an inhaled form. It is then breathed directly into the lungs, where it can act quickly and efficiently at the point where it is most needed. The inhaled form of a bronchodilator will act within one or two minutes. It should be given at the first sign of an attack as these drugs are at their most effective in the earliest stages, before the tubes become blocked with secretions.

Because Sara derived no benefit from either the nebulised Intal or the Alupent syrup, and was rapidly beginning to fit my earlier naïve picture of an 'asthmatic invalid', another drug, Becotide, was now prescribed by the specialist. He did not explain what this was or how it worked, simply that it would 'do her good' and was to be inhaled. The drug is a dry powder contained within a small capsule, which is placed in a 'rotahaler' device (see p. 137) and inhaled through the mouthpiece. Today, Becotide is proving to be an invaluable part of Sara's treatment. She is now seven years old; when Becotide was first prescribed, she was only three. The Becotide rotahaler requires both the ability and the desire to take a deep breath through the mouth, to inhale the powder and then, ideally, the breath should be held for several seconds. Three-year-old Sara hated the sensation of the powder hitting the back of her throat when she breathed it in, and this caused her to be extremely tentative, managing, I'm sure, to swallow more than she inhaled. The doctors at Leeds General Infirmary, by whom she is presently treated, only deemed her old enough at five-and-a-half to handle a rotahaler efficiently—a decision with which I concur totally.

My major grievance regarding this early period of Sara's treatment is that at no time was the function of her various drugs explained to me. I think it is essential that all drugs are not merely prescribed, but have their uses explained both clearly and fully. I believe now that because Sara was unable, at three years old, to inhale both the Intal and the Becotide correctly by the methods prescribed by the specialist, the medications proved totally ineffectual and, consequently, Sara's health showed no signs of improvement whatsoever.

I can think of nothing more distressing than watching a small child growing daily sicker; to consult experts and yet find no solution. Steve and I were by this time quite desperate to find help for Sara. After much soul-searching, we finally decided that the only answer was to take her back to the small Mediterranean island where she had never known any illness. The specialist supported our decision. He felt that the barren, sun-parched land would offer little in the way of allergy-provoking vegetation, and the country was also largely free from any form of chemical pollution in the air, an additional safeguard. This was to prove a sadly incorrect decision on our part. We were so buoyed up by our own expectations, and by the great encouragement which the specialist had given us regarding what he thought would be the 'ideal' conditions prevailing on the island. He had mentioned that a 'change of air' was frequently beneficial to an asthmatic—although he admitted that no one understands why this should be so. What I wish he had told us, since neither Steve nor I realised it at the time, was that, because Sara was still so very sick, despite her various medications and our rigid adherence to her drug 'timetable', her asthmatic condition was still far from being controlled. This was to have extremely distressing consequences for Sara and, as a result, she was to suffer quite dreadfully.

# Chapter Five

Perhaps you also worry that the place where you live may be a contributory factor in your child's asthma, and feel you should move somewhere else. Sara's first specialist was quite right when he talked about a 'change of air' inexplicably being beneficial to an asthmatic; he should have stressed, however, that these improvements are temporary. So, ask yourself whether the stress, expense and inconvenience of the move are going to be worthwhile. Obviously if you live among fields, and hay fever symptoms are a major problem with your child, so that he or she is coughing and wheezing from May to July, you may have good reason to move; otherwise there seems little point. A short holiday is probably a much better idea.

Steve and I spent hours poring over maps after we learned that, far above sea level, say in the dry heights of the Swiss Alps, there is very little incidence of asthma. Nobody seems to know exactly why this should be, but it is certain that there are very few mites found in this extremely dry atmosphere. Obviously this is a somewhat expensive option and, anyway, our coffers were more or less empty after three moves in less than three years. Switzerland was definitely out of the question. So, at the beginning of August 1983, we returned to the island with every expectation of Sara's speedy return to good health. Steve's parents were still living there and were delighted to see us all. They welcomed us into their home and, after all we had told them, were obviously relieved to see Sara looking so much better than they had expected. Once again, she seemed miraculously to have shaken off the constant ill-health and appeared in every way to be a normal, healthy, mischievous child. To start with, all went well; we enjoyed a marvellous trouble-free six-week period in the constant summer sunshine, without the slightest hint of trouble where Sara was concerned. Both James and Sara spent all day, every day, in the swimming pool and Steve and I had no reason not to congratulate ourselves on our decision to return.

After a few weeks, we paid a visit to the family's general practitioner. He did not share our ever-increasing optimism and soon set about dispelling our various illusions. First of all, he was extremely worried to hear that Sara had been diagnosed asthmatic. He had heard from Steve's father that Sara had suffered from frequent bouts of ill-health while she had been living in England, but the cause had never been made clear to him. Had he known the nature of her illness, he would almost certainly have tried to persuade us not to return. He went on to explain that asthma is almost epidemic on the island, although the reason for this is not clear and many different views are put forward. In one attempt to try to control the problem, mimosa and acacia trees, which abound on the island, are being cut down to try to reduce the allergy-related symptoms associated with their pollen. In retrospect, I feel able to pinpoint some of the factors which may have exacerbated Sara's case.

During the reliably settled months of mid June, through July, August and the first couple of weeks in September, the land is indeed arid and largely devoid of any vegetation and its associated allergens. There is little or no wind to whip up the fine particles of dust which Sara, in keeping with most people, and especially her fellow asthmatics, finds particularly irritating. So, during the summer at least, I would expect her to remain healthy in this sort of Mediterranean climate. Even now, however, we must still guard against her dashing about too much, exhausting herself in the scorching, relentless sunshine, as this would cause her to wheeze—but this form of exercise-induced asthma is much easier to predict and so guard against.

The level of humidity on this small island is incredibly high. This is uncomfortable, but not provoking for Sara's asthma in the hot summer months; once the cooler weather sets in, however, the damp seems to permeate everything. This situation can become so acute that total saturation point is almost reached, with levels as high as 94 per cent being recorded. The moisture hangs like a visible curtain of mist in the air. The porous stone, from which the buildings are constructed, acts like a sponge, soaking up the water so that it becomes impossible to remain warm and dry either inside or outside the home. For all those who seek solace in the so-called 'Mediterranean sunshine', take heed of my stepfather's experience when he came out to visit us for a holiday—to enjoy our 'superior' weather conditions in November. He has permanently damaged lungs as an unfortunate consequence of his service in the last war and, far from enjoying any benefit from the promised sunshine, he suffered dreadfully from the all-enveloping damp.

When we had lived previously on the island, I had not been particularly obsessed with the fluctuating weather conditions. However, this time I could not help but notice how Sara had become an accurate human barometer, reflecting the rise and fall of the elements, in the obviously connected improvement and decline of her own health.

Another by-product of damp is mould. I had no idea at the time how provocative this can be to an asthmatic's airways. I knew it was there, of course, but did not realise that mould releases vast quantities of spores into the air. These are very similar to pollen found in flowers, and perform the same function. They are also capable of producing an allergic reaction. Mould is an everyday hazard in such a damp climate, needing as much attention within the home as household dust. It is part of a large group of lower order plants, properly known as fungi. Everywhere on the island some degree of mould was visible in the houses—creeping up from the skirting boards, or down from the ceilings, encircling entrances and running through crevices in the stone-paved floors. The absence of any sort of damp proof course in most, if not all homes fosters the ideal conditions for the powdery-green frostings of mould.

There is yet another thought: perhaps in the cold, damp weather of the winter months Sara spent more time indoors, where she would be exposed continually not only to mould, but to house dust allergies.

I can identify one cause of distress without any hesitation: cold, windy weather. Windy weather conditions seem to be one of the asthmatic's unavoidable hazards. It is true to say that warm winds can carry vast quantities of irritating dust, but the sharp, cold winter winds can provoke an asthmatic's over-sensitive airways almost beyond endurance. Before Sara's asthma was properly controlled, a sudden fierce, cold wind could render her instantly incapable of either speech or breath, as she fought against the spontaneous spasm gripping her airways. All this was induced by the sudden shock of the icy wind entering her lungs. It would be wise to ensure that an asthmatic child does not sleep close to an open window if cold air, pollen or dust could enter unchecked.

I felt sure that the concern of our doctor on the island was misplaced, as Sara had not enjoyed such a run of good health since we had lived there previously; I still felt confident that she could only benefit from our return. The doctor enquired what medications had been prescribed for Sara by the specialist in England, and applauded the use of

Intal—a well-known, safe and uncontroversial preventative medicine. He suggested a simpler and much faster way to administer the drug, which involved dispensing a measured dose from a small aerosol container. My only comment, once again, is that I feel Sara was still too young (just four), to understand fully that she must time her intake of breath to coincide exactly with the sharp pressurised dose as it left the canister. I cannot feel certain that she was deriving any benefit from the medication at this time, and the doctor himself was not at all happy about the use of the drug Becotide in Sara's treatment.

Before I go any further, I must emphasise that Becotide is proving at the present time to be an invaluable part of Sara's treatment, and now that we fully understand the use of this drug and its function, we are quite happy about Sara using it. In 1983, however, we were totally ignorant of the drug's precise nature and only knew that it had been prescribed by the specialist, amongst others, to 'make her better'. The GP was quite mysterious when questioned about his concern. He suggested that we should take his advice and simply throw the capsules away. Naturally, we were rather shocked and pressed him further. He told us, with much reluctance, that Becotide is a steroid medication. To paraphrase a well-known saying and state that, in our case, a little knowledge was a dangerous thing, is rather understating the case; we nearly went mad. How dare anyone prescribe steroids for our daughter without telling us first! Visions of a stunted, muscle-bound, hairy monster, resulting from this unsuspected course of treatment flashed through my furious mind; another clear clarion call for straightforward information to be given by *all* doctors to their patients. I can think of nothing less helpful to all concerned than either indistinct mumblings about steroids, or handing over a prescription without any explanations, so that the patient's own natural curiosity, or that of her parents, leads them to discover that they have been given a drug which they do not understand and one which they believe to be dangerous.

Talking to other parents of asthmatic children, I know that I am not the only person to have regarded steroid therapy as a 'last resort' and one to be avoided at all costs. Nothing frightens people more than the thought of a young child taking or using a steroid medication—and perhaps no other treatment raises so many questions: if my child needs steroids, does it mean that she has severe asthma? Will she always need them and what about the long term effects? They give such wonderful relief, why can we not always use them? And, perhaps the most worrying of all, what about the side effects? On page 134 of Part II of this book, there is a section devoted to steroids as used in the treatment of asthma, which goes into the subject in more detail. This will hopefully not only answer some of the many questions, but will also allay a lot of unnecessary fears.

As far as Sara is concerned, steroids are a major contributory factor in her ability to live a normal life again; you would not want to deny your child that chance. Looking at Sara now gives me all the confidence and proof of success I need, but leaving that doctor's surgery three years ago, it was a different story. We could not wait to get home and throw the 'offending' Becotide capsules down the lavatory!

We continued to stay with Steve's parents throughout the summer, while we continued the search for a suitable home for ourselves. The memories of Sara's asthma drifted further and further behind us, until, suddenly, one evening in late September, the bubble burst. I heard Sara crying out for me from the children's bedroom in the courtyard. I rushed into the room and found her lying across the bed gasping desperately. Helpless tears were running down her fiery cheeks and she could not move towards me or even find enough breath to cry properly. I picked her up and carried her out of the room, across the courtyard to the kitchen, where her grandparents were sitting together chatting. I can remember vividly the shock on their faces when they turned round and, for the first time, saw Sara wheezing. Grandad took her out of my arms and tried to comfort her, but he was soon too upset himself because he just could not do anything for her. The despair you feel when a small child is fighting for breath and fixes her eyes on yours, begging for help, is absolute, because without the necessary medications to hand, you are truly helpless. Our GP proved to be unavailable and so we nursed Sara like a baby for hours, soothing, calming, literally trying to 'love' her better. Very gradually this attack subsided of its own accord and finally, exhausted, Sara fell asleep in my arms.

The following morning I took her in to town to see the doctor. He advised me to continue with the Intal and prescribed some Ventolin syrup, for use at the first sign of a wheeze. As I have mentioned, Ventolin is a bronchodilator, and in syrup form would have a similar effect to the Alupent syrup which had been prescribed on a previous occasion. The doctor expressed the opinion that there was a possibility that Ventolin might be more effective for Sara than Alupent. Inexplicably, the next few weeks were absolutely trouble-free; not a sign of a wheeze. Once again, we began to hope that the attack had been an isolated incident and would not recur. Sara's mood paralleled our own cautious optimism. Overwhelmingly terrified during the course of the attack, she calmed down gradually over the next few days until it seemed that she had not only forgotten the whole incident but, more than that, she behaved as if it had never happened. She never referred to it or questioned me about the mysterious illness which lingered with menacing tenacity in the wings of her life. We all wanted the same simple thing for Sara—please God, let her be well.

On 1st October, 1983, we moved into a beautiful villa in

a quiet country situation. Like most Mediterranean houses, it had cool, marble-floored rooms—a perfect haven, we thought, for the steaming hot summer months. Unfortunately, we had overlooked the fact that there are no clearly defined seasons in the Mediterranean countries. One week the heat is intense, the next can be windy, wet and very cold; the change from summer to winter is abrupt and total. To our dismay, our lovely airy home quickly became a dank, dismal mausoleum. It was soon blindingly obvious that not one room was small enough to be made 'cosy'. Rain lashed down relentlessly from leaden skies, soaking into the sponge-like stone of the villa. The flat roof held a reservoir of puddles which seeped down slowly into the fabric of the building. We bundled ourselves up like polar explorers having discovered that our many radiators were quite useless, due to the many power cuts. Despite the incessant rain, we also began to suffer from regular water shortages. When we questioned the relevant authorities about this unlikely situation, we were informed that there were broken water pipes 'somewhere' between the main supply and ourselves—where, remains one of life's great mysteries! At least our 'glamorous' swimming pool began to earn its keep—as a handy supply of water with which to flush the loo!

We had owned a villa on the island when we lived there before and when the children were babies, but thanks to the archaic but efficient heating system, which heated the whole house from one central flue, we had never experienced bone-chilling conditions like these; I had almost managed to set fire to the house on one occasion, by having the temerity to turn it on full. This situation was quite different—more like trying to make a comfy home inside a cold, wet sponge.

Not surprisingly, everyone's health began to suffer, not least Sara's. Once again the search was on for yet another home. This was a real problem in the winter, when many rental places had been taken off the market. Despite all our efforts to keep Sara as warm and dry as possible, we could see her vitality seeping away from day to day. Eventually, she had to be kept in bed all the time as she became progressively weaker and the all-too familiar cough took yet a firmer grip and gradually, almost imperceptibly, began to take over her life. Soon, her small body was racked continually with the most dreadful coughing fits; some were so severe that tiny blood vessels burst and Sara would scream horribly with revulsion and terror at the sight of the blood she coughed up. Sometimes she was almost past comforting and simply lay steeped in resignation, calling to me over and over again, in a small weary voice, 'Mummy, Mummy, Mummy,' her eyes searching mine for answers, silently begging me to take the hurt away. There were other times when I hardly dared leave her side for a moment, when she sat for hours on end, stiffly upright, supported by a stack of pillows, her arms like two rigid white props, tightly clenched fists rammed deep into the mattress; body arched, head thrown back, as she fought the interminable fight for breath.

Our doctor came every day, sometimes two and three times a day. I know that he tried everything in his power to keep Sara at home with us. No one could be sure just how long this situation would continue. Each day, we looked anxiously for any sign of improvement; it just did not seem possible that Sara could become worse. Some days she seemed a little better, but the recovery was always temporary. We kept a constant watch for any sign of further deterioration, always terrified that we might miss something and find that the attack had worsened beyond our control. Day and night fused into one long vigil but, finally, the doctor said that we really must take her to the hospital. His remedies were exhausted, we were exhausted, and Sara could not carry on at home any longer; she needed more extensive treatment which could only be carried out under hospital supervision and continuous monitoring, which she could only receive in a hospital environment. This was terrible news. We had only kept her at home for so long because the island's hospital had such a bleak and unfriendly reputation; yet we had no alternative. To keep her at home was clearly impossible, so we wrapped her sweat-drenched, panting body in a sheet and set off apprehensively for the hospital.

# Chapter Six

The island's one hospital had an almost Dickensian reputation. It was ringed by high walls, broken only by barriers which were manned by gatemen who were unwelcoming to the point of hostility. We had heard all the rumours about desperate staff shortages and the acute lack of facilities; there was no doubt in either of our minds that this was the sort of place you went to only as the last possible resort. Although it stood only a short distance from our home and the doctor was our personal friend as well as physician, he would not be able to accompany us. Incredible though it may seem, his particular political persuasions, which allied him to the opposition party rather than the ruling government, meant that although he was allowed to practise privately on the island, he was not allowed even to set foot inside the hospital. Obviously many other doctors were in the same position and, in an attempt to fill the huge shortfall of local doctors, their places had been filled with doctors from Eastern bloc countries. Their most out-standing shortfall was their inability to speak the native language. This forced them to converse with the few remaining local doctors and nurses in everyone's second language—English. I had heard about the confusion which resulted from this, but had no idea how many misunder-standings and lost tempers I was due to witness over the next few months.

Steve drove like a man possessed towards the vast hospital complex, for Sara's condition had begun to deteriorate again. Apart from the obvious distress caused by the exhausting, panting wheeze, her overworked lungs were giving her terrible cramp-like pains, which seemed to her to be excruciating stomach ache. Screaming, she curled foetus-like in my arms, until she was completely doubled up with agony. James sat apart from us, frozen, in the furthest corner of the seat, staring fearfully up at his sister; silent in his thoughts, fortunately undemanding, inevitably over-looked. The first frustrating and unnecessary delay came when we reached the front gates. We had virtually to brandish Sara under the nose of the animated uniform standing on guard; eventually we were allowed to pass through. We arrived at Casualty and found it almost empty, apart from one or two lethargic nurses and a couple of scruffy-looking, white-coated individuals, who might or might not have been doctors.

Amazingly, we found that it was impossible to communicate the urgency of Sara's condition; everyone seemed to be both moving and thinking in slow motion. No one responded with the smallest sign of human compassion when confronted by Sara's pitiful condition; instead they told us that we were in the wrong place. We should have been in the children's department, and they gestured vaguely round the corner of the building before returning mechanically to whatever gossip we had so inconsiderately interrupted.

Needless to say, the haphazard directions proved totally inadequate and we lost more time, driving frantically round and round the maze of roads which encompassed the hospital buildings. For all the help she had received so far, I might as well have been standing next to my daughter with my arms tied together, watching her drown. Of course, not understanding Sara's condition properly, or realising that it could deteriorate so rapidly, we had waited far too long before taking her to the hospital—and we were lucky to find someone in time to save her.

At last we found the children's wing and carried Sara inside. After a brief conversation with a nurse, we were shown into a stark room adjoining a ward. A duty doctor arrived, examined Sara and prescribed nebulised Ventolin which they could give her right away. It was incredible how quickly the drug gave her relief. Within a matter of minutes she appeared to recover completely. We were told that we could take her home if we wanted to, although it might be better for her to spend the night in hospital. This seemed a good idea, until we were told that I would not be allowed to stay with Sara. We could pick her up the next day, or, if she stayed any longer than that, we should be allowed to visit her for half-an-hour each day. We were also told not to bring James with us again, as children were not allowed inside the hospital unless they were patients.

All hell broke loose. Sara became hysterical and clung to me, frantically begging me not to leave her. To be honest, there was not the slightest chance of that; I would have been terrified myself at the prospect of being a patient in that unfriendly place. The idea of leaving my own four-year-old sick child there was inconceivable. Our alternative was to return in four hours' time for a further dose of nebulised Ventolin. Steve and I exchanged worried glances. Neither alternative was satisfactory, but the lesser of the two evils would be to take her home. Long before the four hours were up, we could see that she was becoming very sick again. We took her back to the hospital again and this time we had to agree to her admission. Steve returned home with James, who was waiting outside in the car, but I insisted that I should stay with Sara. There were only a few staff present on that Sunday night and they did not give me too much trouble; in the end, I was allowed to remain. Sara was put in a small side ward on her own and I was given a hard, upright chair on which I was prepared to sit all night if necessary—which was just as well, because that is exactly what I did.

We had not been there very long, when a group of nurses came into the room and asked me to leave for a moment while they took Sara's temperature and wrote up her notes. The room being rather small, this seemed a reasonable request, so I agreed to leave. I was surprised when the door was firmly locked behind me. Suddenly, I heard Sara screaming. I banged on the door and shouted for them to let me in. Passing orderlies looked at me with amusement, as if I had gone crazy. Sara's screams went on and on. What on earth were they doing to her? Then the door opened, nurses passed me without a word or a glance, and I barged into the room. Sara had her head turned away from me. She was now attached to a drip and her arm was heavily bandaged to hold it in position. When the drip was later removed and the bandages taken away, I was able to see from the extensive bruising and many tiny wounds, just how many attempts it had taken the inept nurses to insert the needle.

During the next few hours Sara's breathing eased, but she seemed to be in a state of shock. For a long time she lay quite still, staring silently at the wall, refusing to look at me. I had unwittingly betrayed her and failed her for the first time. Finally she slept. I did not.

The grey dawn brought the soft, padding feet and low murmurs of nurses on the new shift. Curious groups paused outside the door to stare in at us, and I had the distinct impression that I was an unprecedented intruder in their domain. Sara woke slowly, with a careful hesitancy, as if examining every detail of her confinement before determining the best way to cope with it. The drip was thankfully still secure in her small bandage swathed arm, which was secured to a splint; this in its turn was fastened down to the bed on which she lay. She still drew away from me and responded to my attention with only mechanical obedience. I wished I could do something positive for her, but at least I had been right in my insistence to remain with her. During the night I had seen a small child brought into the next room. She, too, had needed a drip and, through the glass panel which divided us, I saw her struggling and screaming with fright. Rather than trying to soothe her fears for even a moment, I saw the nurses quickly tie her arms and legs to the bed with bandages, and then they left her whimpering pitifully in the dark room, quite alone.

I shall never forget the heavy silence which consumed that neglected ward; crying had undoubtedly proved a pointless exercise. Then, I remember, a door opened suddenly at the end of the gloomy, mustard-glossed corridor and a doctor swept in, flanked by a bustling group of students. I was about to meet the doctor who, one day, would not only save my daughter's life but would also be responsible for restoring my rapidly diminishing faith in the medical profession. Why was he different? Perhaps his compassion was the key. If you cannot feel the suffering of others as your own remembered pain, then you become simply a well-programmed machine, capable of spewing out prescriptions and tonics, but never truly knowing the gift of healing. From the moment he sat down on Sara's bed and took her hand in his, both Sara and I began to gain confidence. Unfortunately, a representative from the hospital's administrative staff chose this moment to put in an appearance and insisted that I leave immediately—as my presence in the hospital was against regulations. The doctor was in the frustrating position of being a British specialist on secondment to the hospital's Paediatric Department, and so lacking any real authority. Despite his patient and lengthy attempts to persuade this person that my leaving might seriously prejudice the condition of his patient, I was told over and over again, as if by a robot, to leave, as if he did not hear what the doctor was saying. Although I was desperately reluctant to leave Sara, I decided that, rather than subject her to an unpleasant scene, which was the way things were developing, I had better go.

When Steve and I returned for the permitted half-hour visit in the afternoon, the same doctor was waiting for us at the door to the ward. He told us that as Sara's condition was now stabilised, we could take her home immediately. We were a little surprised by this and asked him whether she would be all right at home. 'You don't want her in this place,' was his reply.

Steve swept Sara up in his arms and carried her down the stairs to the car. The very first thing she wanted, apart from a cheese sandwich, was to see James again. James was still only three and had been left hurriedly with Steve's parents. I felt guilty, knowing that he was bewildered and unhappy, wondering where we were and why there was so little time for him in our lives. It was very touching to see him toddling across the courtyard towards us and the two children then clinging to each other, hugging and kissing. How good it felt to be together again.

We were overdue for some good news, but we were about to be rewarded. Steve had not wasted a moment during the short time Sara had been in hospital; he had found us a better place to live—a modern apartment on the seafront. We both felt sure that it would have many advantages. It was in the centre of town, very close to our doctor, and felt both warm and dry—although we were now well into the bitterly cold winter season. Even the doctor thought the situation ideal: we were well away from any potentially allergenic vegetation and the compact apartment would be so much easier to keep warm than the rambling villa.

Sara was now taking Ventolin tablets regularly, rather than waiting for an attack to manifest itself, and these were in a much stronger dose than the syrup which she had taken previously. We also maintained the regular doses of Intal. We asked our doctor about the advisability of buying a nebuliser to use at home, and he told us that neither the nebuliser nor the Ventolin solution to use in it was available to the public on the island's home market. This did not pose too much of a problem as Steve travelled frequently to the UK where both were readily obtainable. Our GP still was not keen on the idea—possibly because Sara's condition was extremely unpredictable and could worsen very rapidly. Whatever his reason, he asked us to wait a little longer to 'see what happens'. Our inexperience urged us to caution and so we agreed.

How easy it is to be wise in retrospect. I have simply lost count now of the number of potentially unpleasant attacks which we have managed to avert by giving Sara her pre-scribed dose of Ventolin in our own nebuliser, 'at the first sign of a squeak'. Unfortunately, it was to be many months and many hospital admissions later before we took matters into our own hands and bought our cherished nebuliser. To feel that at last you have some control over the situation and can probably avoid a distressing attack, is the most wonderful feeling of release. Confidence floods back, both for parent and child, when relief is there, immediately to hand. Now we have not one, but two nebulisers: an electric model for home use, and a foot pump model, which proves invaluable in the most unlikely situations—on aeroplanes, boats, beside swimming pools, on the beach and in the car. Sara never travels without her nebuliser and does not think twice about using it; the difference it has made to her life is beyond reckoning.

It may be possible in some cases to have the use of a nebuliser in your own home, free of charge. Make enquiries at your local hospital or doctor's surgery.

# Chapter Seven

I noticed a pattern evolving with Sara's health, which gradually became clear to me following her first experience as a patient in the island's hospital. During the week following her discharge she became steadily stronger, her breathing quite normal, and the cough diminished daily until, by the second week, she was apparently quite well—no cough, wheeze, lethargy, or anything at all which might cause concern. Then, just as our confidence was beginning to return, she hit the downward slope. Almost imperceptibly at first, the symptoms returned. First, a lot of throat clearing and grumpiness, then the cough—just the odd one to start with, so that you heard it and worried momentarily before forgetting all about it. By the start of the third week we were unable to ignore the fact that Sara was heading for trouble again. During the next four months she was admitted to hospital every three weeks. The attacks became progressively more severe and her deterioration at the onset of each attack more rapid.

In between her hospital admissions Sara was attending as an outpatient. More skin tests were suggested. I was sceptical with regard to their reliability but, at the same time, desperate to clutch at any straw. We arrived to find approximately ten other children lined up to have skin tests with Sara. As soon as Sara saw the pin scratching the first child, she screamed, clung to me and refused to allow the doctor to touch her. I was filled with totally irrational impatience and frustration; far from feeling any compassion for Sara, I could have struck her. Thankfully, I did not, but I just could not allow myself to believe that we were never going to find an answer. How could I explain to a little girl that a few more 'pricks' in her arm might, and only might, be the means of ensuring that she would never again have to suffer a drip in her arm in hospital, when, to Sara, one needle looked much like another?

The move to the apartment had not helped Sara at all; she coughed convulsively, all night long. Now we were faced with the additional problem of complaints from our neighbours that Sara's cough was keeping them awake. How could we explain to them what we could not understand ourselves? Why could the doctors not stop Sara coughing? What were we to do next? We had not simply moved house several times, we had moved countries. We had visited numerous doctors, none of whom had been able to provide any long-term relief for Sara, and the best they could offer us was that one day she might grow out of it. How was Sara, and, indeed, how were we all, supposed to get on with our lives in the meantime?

During these four months, Sara was hardly ever well long enough to be able to attend school. The few times we were able to leave the apartment it seemed that the cough returned with force. 'Fancy letting that child out with such a dreadful cough', seemed to have become an inevitable remark on each such expedition.

Occasionally, we managed to avoid a hospital admission by taking her along to the ward, where they would give Sara nebulised Ventolin; she would then return home and our doctor called in each day to supervise a course of steroid tablets. On the occasions when she had to be admitted to the hospital, she was also given steroid tablets and, if the attacks were particularly serious, which usually they were, steroids were given through a drip. As the attacks were so close together, these high-dose courses of steroids were becoming almost consecutive and, as a consequence, some side effects from the steroids were now becoming apparent. Sara had become considerably over-weight, in fact she weighed more then, when she was four years old than she does now she is eight. Her face, naturally round and chubby, became unpleasantly bloated or 'moon faced'. My once bright, happy child, had become morose, whiny and difficult—who could blame her?

All Sara's hospital admissions at this time were extremely unpleasant and traumatic events. Every sick child needs the comfort and reassurance which only her parents can supply; who more than an asthmatic child, whose very condition can be exacerbated by emotional upsets? Yet half-an-hour a day was all the time I was permitted to stay with her. Believe it or not, the ward door was actually locked until the bell rang for visiting time, and was locked again behind us as we parents trooped out obediently at the end of visiting time; what a place to leave a child! To make matters worse, Steve still had to travel extensively and, oddly enough, Sara's hospital admissions seemed to coincide with his trips out of the country. Steve's parents lived a considerable distance away from us and I was frequently at a loss over where to leave James on the occasions when it became necessary to take Sara to the hospital—sometimes at a moment's notice. Once, in desperation, I left James with our maid, a pleasant young girl with children of her own. She told me later that James cried inconsolably the whole time I was away from him, and asked the girl repeatedly to please take him home. When her husband arrived back from work, James tried again: 'Will you take me home to my mummy?' The man tried to placate James by telling him that it was raining heavily and he would take him home later. James was not to be so easily discouraged. He gathered up his small anorak and stood waiting by the door until I returned, tears pouring silently down his face.

One dark, wet evening in March 1984, Sara became very

sick, very quickly. Steve was away and totally out of reach, except by the factory telex, as he was visiting a 'Rig Camp' in the desert regions of North Africa. Within minutes rather than hours Sara was wheezing frantically. There was no time for a telephone call to Steve's parents or to make any other arrangements; I had no alternative but to take James along with us in the car, even though I knew he would not be allowed inside the hospital. Sara was unable to stand and was terribly heavy, but somehow I managed to carry her down three flights of stairs before dashing back for James. 'Sara's sick,' he said softly. I often smile to myself when people discuss with pride their toddler's early words; I can only hope James has forgotten his.

The only sound in the car on the mad dash to the hospital was Sara's wheeze. It did not seem possible that any air at all could be finding its way through the river of mucus to her lungs. The horrible pumping rhythm of viscid bubblings seemed far too dreadful to be real.

Occasionally, I was able to glance over and see Sara barely conscious, and James sitting mute with misery and confusion. We arrived at the barriers at the entrance to the hospital, where I gave a barely civil explanation while the man peered into the car, before I accelerated away to the Casualty Department; even though Sara was a regular patient, we were never able to take a short cut and head straight for the ward. First she had to be examined, diagnosed and the relevant documents completed before they would allow her to be treated on the ward. I carried her into Casualty, having no alternative but to leave James in the car. There appeared to be some sort of evening surgery being conducted in the Casualty Department; the whole place was packed with people and was very, very hot. Everyone seemed to be talking at once in their own language and the only available nursing staff were already besieged by crowds of people. There was nowhere to sit or put Sara down, and no wheelchairs. As I still had her in my arms, I could not get through the crowds to attract the attention of a nurse. I looked at her and knew that, although in some ways she might appear to be recovering, the fact that her breathing was quieter did not herald an improvement. It was very shallow and rapid; she was not sleeping quietly in my arms, she was unconscious.

The sweat was pouring off me as I stood uncertainly, holding Sara, in the middle of this mad-house. Then, taking myself by surprise more than anyone else, I charged. Using my best Joyce Grenfell voice, which brooked no argument, I declaimed, 'Out of my way. This child is very sick.' Whereupon I strode straight into the consultant's office.

My sudden appearance with Sara was greeted in stony silence. Various degrees of alarm and indignation registered on the faces of the doctors, nurses, patient and other assorted supernumeraries. I ignored the ensuing uproar as the room erupted, and took Sara to the examination couch where I laid her down and waited. Everyone had apparently forgotten us in their pressing need to vocalise their outrage at my obviously unprecedented intrusion. Finally a doctor noticed us, came over and examined Sara briefly. His broken English was extremely sketchy, but he made himself clear enough as he began berating the nearest nurse for not bringing us straight in to him. He cleared the room and told me that Sara was suffering from pleurisy and should be admitted to hospital immediately. Sick as she undoubtedly was, this piece of information communicated itself to Sara. She was plainly terrified and began crying, 'Mummy, Mummy,' and clinging to me like a little limpet. I tried to explain to the doctor that she was in fact an asthmatic and that she had been a patient at the hospital before. He did not appear to understand me and persisted in disagreeing with what I told him, instructing me brusquely to take her to the children's ward. Everyone scurried around trying to look efficient, but no one could find a stretcher, so I was told to carry her.

I lugged poor Sara off the couch and pushed my way out through the crowds. It seemed very quiet outside by the car after the mayhem in the Casualty Department. James, displaying his usual self-possession, had switched on the interior lights of the car and was playing quietly with his toys on the back seat; I was very proud of him.

I parked outside the children's ward and again, having no alternative, left James alone in the car while taking Sara inside. The foreign doctor was waiting for us. Sara, still barely conscious but sounding now like a furious steam engine, was flailing around, no doubt as a result of an extreme lack of oxygen. I felt monstrous letting them take her out of my arms as her tiny hands groped feebly to cling on to me. 'She will have to be sedated.' I could not believe my own ears. The doctor was prescribing a sedative for Sara—surely the most dangerous course of action possible for a child in the middle of a severe asthma attack. Anyone could see she was almost incapable of breathing at all, and yet the doctor was now advocating a course of treatment which would inevitably suppress her breathing still further. 'You'll have to move your car.' Voices from a nightmare, and yet all this was actually happening. Blast the car, they could tow it away, but No! What about James? I was almost hysterical by now. I was not allowed into the room where they had taken Sara, and was desperate to find help. I fled from that hospital, frantic, with a very real fear that they might kill my little girl.

I drove away, crying, but I had to force myself to consider objectively what I should do. It was pointless approaching our GP, as he would not be allowed to interfere with the treatment of any patient within the hospital; it was too late to try to find someone who might possibly be able to give me the address of the one doctor at the hospital who seemed fully to understand Sara's condition; and there was also James to consider. I reached a decision and drove to the home of some friends of ours who were islanders themselves. Our friendship had previously been on a fairly superficial social level; now it was the middle of the night and I needed their help badly.

Whatever assistance I had anticipated as I drove to their house was supplied tenfold. Within minutes of our arrival everything was in hand. James was quickly settled into their own bed and I was speeding back to the hospital with my friend's husband. We found Sara in an oxygen tent, surrounded by tubes and drips. The ward was very cold and she felt frozen. There was not a scrap of bedding on her bed, not even a pillow. She was dressed only in her pants, and her feet especially were like little blocks of ice. My friend went to find a nurse and, miraculously, bedding appeared, even a pair of woolly bedsocks. We covered her carefully and were relieved to see that she was sleeping peacefully. We were told that there would be no doctors available who were familiar with Sara's case until the following morning's round at 8 a.m.

The nurse seemed almost eager to confide in my friend, her fellow countryman, and further probing revealed that Sara's condition had become so critical following the treatment by the 'Eastern bloc' doctor, that the ward sister had been forced to rouse the head of the Paediatric Department from his bed; this gentleman had left Sara only moments before we arrived. The nurse promised to telephone if there was any change in Sara's condition and, as she was still fast asleep and breathing quietly I was persuaded to leave.

When we returned, my friends insisted that I should share their bedroom with James, and it was only some time later that I learned that they had dozed on and off all night in their children's room, taking it in turns to ring the hospital every hour.

This time Sara's return to strength was slow. She had to stay in the hospital for more than a week. The factory had managed to contact Steve by telex in the desert camp, but he was forced to endure an unbearable delay as he waited for the company plane to fly him to the nearest international airport; the service was only operated once a week in that remote area. Each day I geared myself up to run the gauntlet of the gatemen before being allowed inside the hospital grounds. Then I had to wait outside the locked ward with numerous other anxious parents before being allowed in for the precious half-hour's visit; there was barely time to hold Sara and talk to her before I was thrown out again. She told me that as soon as I left, all the toys and presents I took for her were taken away and only returned when visiting time came round again. The nurses teased her particularly over her beloved panda from which she was never separated. They snatched it from her and played catch with it over her head, laughing at her pleas to return it. I tried to feed her for the day, too, as I had occasionally caught sight of the slop she was expected to eat. I 'rented' space in the ward's fridge, and always took the precaution of ensuring that there was enough for the staff as well.

During this awful week I had my one and only accident with the car, when I knocked a man off his motorbike. My whole concentration had become centred on Sara to the exclusion of everything else. Fortunately it was only a nudge at our local garage, and the man was unhurt, although at the time he was obviously having difficulty deciding how many of the numerous bumps on his decrepit old machine I could be held responsible for. Luckily for me we had a good account at the garage, and several oily mechanics persuaded him to overlook the incident.

Sara's homecoming coincided with Steve's return from his trip. The tension abounding in our apartment now was a very real threat to the well-being of us all. Sara had to stay in bed and rest, so that she would not run around and possibly risk tiring herself, which might have precipitated another attack. She was quite well enough, however, to be a little tyrant when it came to demanding constant stimulus and amusement. James was fretful and naughty by turns as he played for my attention. Steve was both exhausted by his work and frustrated by his inability to set our lives on an even keel, torn as he was between his necessary business commitments, which provided our comfort and security, and his desire to be with us at this time when we all plainly needed him so very badly. Wherever he turned he found himself in the wrong place.

Sara was still coughing during the night, and I had to let Steve sleep to ensure that he would be fit for his work in the morning. I stayed up with Sara and marvelled at her capacity to be alert, bright and ever-demanding the following day. Finally, I was forced to admit that I did not possess her boundless vitality and was more or less worn out. We decided to ask my mother whether she would fly out from England to lend a hand. When she arrived, we organised a shift system, whereby I would stay up all night if necessary, and she would then do the day shift, caring for and playing with both children so that I could get some sleep at last.

In many ways this eased the situation enormously, although for the first time Steve and I were finding time to talk about our deepest fears. We realised that we were reaching a point where it was no longer possible for Sara to live on the island where the medical facilities were plainly inadequate as far as she was concerned. Steve could not contemplate leaving the business so soon, as he had only just begun to see signs of a revival in the factory following his return. To leave now would totally demoralise the workforce and undoubtedly mean our losing everything he had worked so very hard to rebuild.

That the business could not survive without him travelling extensively to clinch the major contracts, and then returning to supervise their completion in person, had been proved without a doubt when we had previously moved to England. I had to face the fact that I could not remain on the island with the children. We discussed our position continually, but could find no happy solution. In the end we agreed to give our family life together one more chance, in the forlorn hope that Sara might miraculously recover. In retrospect, it seems futile and even pathetic, but who could blame us?

It was my mother who persuaded us both to take a long weekend away from the situation. Knowing that she was the one person I would trust to take on the responsibility of Sara's care in my stead, we agreed to fly to London for a short rest. We arranged for the GP to call at the apartment twice a day while we were away, and the friends with whom I had stayed while Sara was in hospital offered to call in every day. My mother had the use of my car and so we did several 'dry runs' to the hospital to ensure that she was fully acquainted with the route, just in case.

It was almost impossible to unwind in the short time we could bear to be away. The office called daily with their ever-present list of urgent problems, and I spent a lot of time ringing the apartment to reassure myself that all was well. I felt happy when I spoke to my mother and the children, who seemed to thrive on her company, as indeed they might, although I am sure that my tension must have communicated itself to them and made them apprehensive in turn. The luxury of uninterrupted sleep was one gift I could not overlook and, even after two or three nights, I felt wonderfully refreshed. By the end of our stay I felt almost normal again.

# Chapter Eight

We returned to find that life at the apartment had not been without its dramas. My mother had considerately resisted the temptation to tell me that James had wrenched the small stepladder from its cupboard, propped it up against the hall fitment and climbed up it until he could scramble up the shelves. This had enabled him to reach the supposedly 'child-proof' cupboard where I kept Sara's pills, some six feet off the floor. He had then emptied all the tubs of pills and capsules onto the floor. Mother, hearing the rumpus, arrived in time to find him sitting on the floor, happily building towers with the numerous containers. The pills and capsules were lying discarded all around him. Terrified that he might have had time to sample some of the medications, she bundled Sara and James into the car to take him to the hospital for a check-up. Fortunately, our friends chose just this moment to arrive for their daily visit. They drove my ashen-faced mother and children to the hospital, where they all experienced for themselves the incredible disorganisation of the reception area at Casualty. Incredibly, it seemed that the clerk on duty was barely literate. He struggled endlessly to write down the few particulars, until finally our friends grabbed the form from him in frustration and filled it out for him. They apologised to my mother for what they saw as a shaming incident, and assured her that even these minor government appointments were obtained through political favour rather than aptitude. Eventually, James was examined by a doctor, who thankfully found no sign of his having swallowed any of the medications.

Soon after our return, my mother had to return home to England. Steve and I were no closer to any kind of acceptable solution and were resigned to living on an emotional tight-rope, constantly hoping that the inevitable would not happen. James was able now to attend a small local kindergarten. He seemed to be enjoying the change, especially as it entailed a coach ride in the school transport with his favourite teacher. I was free to look after Sara and help her to catch up with all the school work she had missed due to her illness. Occasionally, she was well enough to attend the local convent school. I say 'occasionally', as only two weeks were to pass between her discharge from hospital and her first visit to Outpatients. During these two weeks there had been good days and bad, but neither were predictable or accountable. Steve decided to attend Outpatients with us; he felt we must make a concerted effort this time to see exactly what could be done for Sara.

The waiting-room was packed and we were relieved to be the first in the queue. Sara was very pale, but quite perky, as we sat waiting for the doctor to arrive. She was looking forward to seeing him again; he was the one doctor in whom we all had so much faith and Sara simply adored him. He arrived and we were ushered into his room. We had planned to wait until he completed his examination before plunging into our many questions regarding the prospects for Sara's return to good health. Her breathing certainly appeared normal enough to us, and there were none of the usual warning signs: lethargy, coughing, throat-clearing. The doctor's examination did not take any longer than usual, but rather than laughing and joking with her as he usually did, he became very quiet and thoughtful. He sat Sara down on top of his desk and perched on his chair, holding her hands in his.

'What is it? What's wrong?' we asked him. He asked us to bear with him for a while. He told us that there was nothing wrong at that moment, but he did not want us to take Sara home. At the same time he knew what a trauma it was for Sara every time she was admitted to the hospital. 'Please wait for a while, I'm not happy,' he said in the understated way he needed to adopt if Sara was not to be alarmed. He told a nurse to go and inform the other patients that there would be a considerable delay, and that those who could should make alternative appointments for the next clinic. Steve and I exchanged frightened glances and sat silently, waiting to see what would happen. The doctor sat quietly, absorbed with Sara as they drew pictures together and chattered chummily about this and that. Occasionally he would casually take her wrist and feel her pulse, and once or twice he asked her if she would mind if he had 'another little listen' to her chest.

Unbelievably, we sat in his room for almost an hour until he said, 'I'm sorry; she must be admitted.' Sara protested louder than usual, no doubt relying on Daddy to protect her. There still did not seem to be very much to be alarmed about; certainly, had she been at home, I would not have thought it necessary to bring her to the hospital, but the doctor's intuition told him that we were about to encounter an attack more severe than either Steve or I could have anticipated. Steve pleaded with him to change his mind; the thought of admitting Sara yet again was terrible. The doctor understood and sympathised with our apprehension, but insisted that we had no alternative. Steve made it clear that if Sara was to be admitted, then I would stay with her. Whatever strings he must pull would be pulled, and at whatever cost.

The doctor instructed the nurse to prepare the necessary forms for him to sign and told us not to worry, as he would come with us to the ward in order to explain the special nature of Sara's condition to the sister in charge.

Despite the fact that this must have brought Sara's hospital admissions on the island well into double figures, incredibly it was the first time Steve had been with me since that first occasion. I can truthfully say that I was more than happy to be able to hand over both the carrying and the brunt of the organisation to him.

When we arrived at the ward, the doctor, himself a foreigner as far as the staff were concerned, being, as I have said, on secondment from Britain to the Paediatric Department, was placed in the unlikely position of practically having to beg for a private room for his patient. Sara still did not outwardly appear to be sick and the nurses' disapproval of his request was made all too obvious. I could not help but recall a previous occasion, when a junior nurse had tried to turn me away from the ward, even though the Casualty doctor had issued a form to say that Sara must be admitted for treatment. 'There doesn't look much wrong with her; it must be a mistake,' she had said. This time our doctor cajoled, while Steve threatened, dropping every politically favoured name he could dredge up. Begrudgingly, we were eventually allocated a small room 'round the corner, where no one would see us'. This seemed unlikely, but we did not wait to argue the point.

We settled Sara down in bed. Although she was still quite cheerful, knowing that I would not be leaving her this time, I noticed that she had developed a slight wheeze. I was not worried, in fact I felt quite confident. After all, what better place for her than hospital, even this one? I felt absolutely certain that the attack had been caught in its initial stages, and prompt treatment would now abort it before it had a chance to develop.

Steve left the room to go and telephone his parents, to warn them that he would be arriving with James as soon as the morning school closed. The doctor came into the room and examined Sara again. He was very gentle with her and, talking quietly, asked her not to be frightened but she must have the drip again and an oxygen tent. The very mention of the drip rendered her rigid with terror. 'No, Mummy, no!' she cried, her eyes boring into mine, eloquent with despair. I held her close and tried to say something to comfort her. I felt numb and sick as I whispered meaningless platitudes and necessary lies into her tangled hair. 'It won't hurt. Just a little prick. Then you'll be better.' The doctor told me that I would have to leave the room while they inserted the drip, and it took two nurses to prise Sara from me. I was given no alternative other than to stand outside the door listening to her screams.

Steve returned and we were both allowed back into Sara's room. She was beyond misery. I sat by her bed, holding her hand, and her eyes did not leave mine for a moment. How I wished that I could will some of my own strength into her. Steve said that he must get back to the office, but would return in an hour or so. So we sat, Sara and I, waiting for the relief which always came very quickly after she was receiving medication through the drip. I soon noticed with concern that, rather than easing, her breathing was becoming more distressed. Within minutes she had developed a blue tinge around her mouth, and even the fingernails on the little hand clutching my own had turned an ominous smutty colour. I rang for the nurse who looked at Sara and then raced out of the room. The doctor returned with the ward sister and more nurses. The room filled up as they circled Sara's bed. More drugs were injected into the tubing of the drip. Sara had become extremely restless, although she was still clinging to my hand. Her breathing had become so rapid it hardly seemed possible that a child's body could cope with the demands of her lungs. She jerked so uncontrollably that the drip was wrenched out of her arm. No one had time to ask me to leave the room this time as the doctor and nurses fought to reinsert the needle. Sara's strength was formidable as her body bucked violently.

I ran out of the room and telephoned James's school, the factory and Steve's parents; he was somewhere in between. Whoever saw him first must send him straight back to the hospital—something was very wrong.

I raced back into Sara's room. Another doctor had been called. Everyone was talking at once. A man's voice shouted, 'Open the windows! Someone clear this room!' My only thought was Sara, to touch her, hold her. Her appearance appalled me. She was grey, clammy, only her eyes seemed normal as she felt for my hand and stared frantically up at me. 'Help me, Mummy,' she gasped, 'I can't breathe!' I have never felt so impotent.

Steve returned and the doctor ushered us both out of the room. It was almost impossible to concentrate on his words. Sara was screaming for me like a wounded animal as the nurses tried to insert yet another drip. Even the doctor was distracted and left us in mid-sentence to go and insert the needle himself. Steve looked bemused, his face waxen. 'What's happening?' he asked me. The doctor came out at last and told us that Sara was desperately ill and must be transferred to the intensive treatment unit immediately. We followed him mutely to the desk where he made the necessary telephone call. I did not take in his words but certainly the tone of his voice fully conveyed the urgency of Sara's case . . . and yet, there seemed to be a problem. His face was grim as he turned to us. There were no beds available in the Intensive Care Unit.

'Mr Sutherland, Mr Sutherland!' The doctor gripped Steve's arm fiercely and spoke slowly and clearly as if to a small child. 'If you know someone, someone who can help us, please, call him now.' He thrust the telephone into Steve's hand. The meaning was clear enough. Steve dialled the one person who could help us. Within minutes of putting the telephone down, it rang. The doctor answered. A bed was available for Sara in the Intensive Care Unit. The man Steve had called was an acquaintance who wielded considerable influence within the ruling political party.

Moments later we were rushing behind the trolley as it carried Sara down the maze of passages which led to the unit. Steve and I were stopped at the reception area while the doctor hastily donned a gown, mask and covers for his shoes. The unit's nurses were already waiting outside for Sara and she disappeared through the swing doors. We were told to sit down and wait as the doctor hurried after her. Again the screams, over and over 'Mummy, Mummy, Mummy!' Where did she find the strength? Two more doctors dashed into the unit and grabbed gowns from the rack. Then silence.

We sat, frozen, searching the silence for some indication of what might be happening beyond the doors. A young doctor came out. We both stood up. 'Are you the little girl's parents?' We said we were and the doctor asked us if we would like to see Sara. He asked us not to let her see us, as it was imperative that they kept her calm. We donned robes and followed him into the unit, dreading what we might find. Sara was in an area separate from the main body of the unit; we were able to see her by peeping round the curtains of the small room. She was naked and propped up in the bed, lost in the midst of machinery and monitors, wires and tubes everywhere. I noticed that she appeared to be sitting up by herself and took this to be a good sign, but the doctor dispelled my illusions. He explained that her position was the one usually adopted by someone desperate for oxygen. She was indeed bolt upright, head thrown back, ribs prominent, chest pumping furiously. 'Can you make sure the drip stays in position now?' I asked, remembering the screams. The doctor told me that Sara now had a 'long-line' drip in position, and that she would be unable to pull it out. I paled at the thought of that being inserted into her arm while she was still fully conscious. Sara's doctor caught sight of us and left her side. He ushered us out again into the reception area and told us that his major worry was that Sara might need ventilating; the hospital's machine had never been used on a child before. Everything humanly possible had been done for Sara, there was nothing more that they could do. He told us as gently as he could that she had a 50/50 chance of surviving the attack and suggested that we go home and pray.

How I envied our friends their faith. Word spreads swiftly on a small island and, even as we arrived at Steve's father's house, the calls were coming in. Catholic friends were visiting a famous shrine to pray for Sara; Quaker friends were holding a meeting of their healing group; the nuns at the convent school were praying. Only Steve and I felt numb and useless. A lifetime of agnosticism does not lend itself well to these occasions. I tried, we both tried. In such desperation, who else is there to turn to but God?

# Chapter Nine

When we arrived back at Steve's parents' to see James and decide what to do next, we found that there was a previously planned dinner party in full swing. We shut ourselves away in the study to avoid the possibility of questions which we just could not answer. James had been put to bed and was thankfully fast asleep. We endured an agonising wait before calling the hospital. When we telephoned the unit we were told that Sara was 'very poorly', and that they would call us immediately if there was any change in her condition. This was not good enough. No discussion was necessary between us. We left the house immediately and returned to the hospital.

We were not allowed to go into the Intensive Care Unit, but were relieved to find that Sara's doctor was still there. He came out to see us as soon as he heard that we had arrived. He reiterated his opinion that there was nothing to be gained by our being there at this time. There was nothing at all we could do for Sara and he suggested quite forcibly that we should now go home and rest in case we were needed later; he gave us his assurance that he would ring us personally should the need arise. We felt totally useless and utterly despondent as we drove home. We left James at Steve's parents' and sat up together all night at the apartment, waiting for the telephone call which, thankfully, never came.

At 8 a.m. we returned apprehensively to the hospital. Sara's condition had stabilised but only during the last few grey hours of dawn. It transpired that her doctor had been at Sara's bedside all through the night, her condition had been so critical. This was all the more remarkable as we discovered that he had to leave the island that day to attend a medical conference in Washington, USA; he must have been completely exhausted. He passed Sara's case on to two senior consultants, as she was to stay in the hospital for another ten days. However absorbed this man must have been in his medical conference, he still cared enough to find time to write to me about Sara, telling me of his concern for her and sending his good wishes for her recovery.

Before he left the island, this same doctor somehow managed to dictate a letter of referral to a chest specialist in London. He told us that, in his opinion, the medical facilities on the island were totally inadequate for a child like Sara; we must take her home to Britain, perhaps for good. The consequences for us as a family did not bear thinking about. We arranged that the moment Sara was discharged from the hospital we would fly home with her to see the specialist.

Although deemed fit to travel, the specialist in London found that Sara was still suffering from bronchopneumonia. Fortunately, we still owned the house in Yorkshire and would be able to take the children there for Sara's recuperative period. As well as antibiotics, the specialist prescribed a drug new to us, Theophylin. This came in the form of capsules which worked on a twelve-hour slow-release principle. Theophylin is a bronchodilator and the two twelve-hourly doses ensured that she received the benefit of the drug continuously around the clock. We purchased our own nebuliser in order to be able to administer a solution of Intal which the specialist felt would be a foolproof method of administering the drug.

This Sara was to inhale four times a day. Before we left him, the specialist echoed my own thoughts when he remarked that it was a great pity that, in many instances, patients must endure what amounts to an apprenticeship of suffering before their condition receives the serious attention it merits.

We returned to Yorkshire, Sara's next appointment having been set for two weeks' time. Once again Steve was forced to leave us and return to his business responsibilities on the island.

Everything about the day when I was due to take Sara back to see the specialist in London was lousy. Bundled up against the dank, freezing-cold day, we still shivered as we stood on the platform waiting for the train. I had been assured that the early morning commuter train was never late and so felt justified in choosing that form of travel. The train was more than an hour behind schedule and we had a mad dash to get to the specialist in time for Sara's appointment. At first she seemed fine, full of energy and extremely alert, but while we were discussing her various medications I was alarmed to notice that she had suddenly become very drowsy. She climbed up onto my knee and, although it was still early in the afternoon, she fell deeply asleep. This had always proved in the past to be a warning sign, and I voiced my fears to the specialist. I emphasised that this sort of unusual behaviour had preceded several severe attacks.

He called for a thermometer and examined Sara again, briefly but thoroughly. I was surprised that he did not express any concern at the fact that he was able to move her around quite considerably during the course of his examination, and yet not once did she wake from her unnaturally deep sleep. I explained that we had a long train journey ahead of us and I was apprehensive at the thought of being out of reach of medical assistance for several hours. Sara was so unusually pale and still that I was rather hoping that he might suggest admitting her for observation to one of his wards at the hospital, which was only across the road from his consulting room. I was to be disappointed. Carrying Sara, I was politely but firmly ushered out of his office. Moments later, he hurried out, obviously late for his next appointment. Whether it would simply have been too much trouble for a man in a hurry to take more precautions with a child already recognised as being at risk, I shall never know.

A sympathetic receptionist called a taxi for me. Sara had not stirred in my arms; I had no idea how we were going to make it back to Leeds. When I arrived at the station, still carrying my sleeping child, I staggered off in search of our train. Worse was to come. Our reserved seats in the second class compartment had been double-booked and I was unable to find a single empty seat the whole length of the train. Sara was now wheezing and I was unable to carry her a step further, so I braved the wrath of the guard and commandeered a vacant first class carriage. We still had a three-hour journey to face before I could take her to a hospital. There was no alternative, I just had to sit it out and hope for the best. I cursed that consultant ferociously during our endless journey, as Sara lay panting in my arms. I had plenty of time to reflect that this was one occasion when there was little satisfaction in being able to say to that learned and highly respected man, 'I told you so'.

Fortunately my mother met the train. She was as distressed as I was to see Sara so sick again. We raced off to the Casualty Department at Leeds General Infirmary, where Sara was admitted immediately. I am afraid that my attitude towards the doctor in Casualty was something more than brusque; I was still seething at the consultant's lack of perception and concern. It seemed to me that this eminent gentleman was in as much of a hurry to 'be done' with his patient as he was to present his not inconsiderable bill.

The duty doctor was actually extremely gentle and sympathetic. Despite Sara's previous horrific experiences in hospital, she barely flinched when he inserted the needle for the drip. Perhaps she was past caring, but I like to think she may have been responding co-operatively to the doctor's kindness. Sara was placed on my knee and we were both whisked by wheelchair to the children's ward. She was settled in bed very quickly and 'plugged in' to the drip—the attachment was already firmly bandaged to her arm extending from the needle which had been inserted in Casualty, so no traumas whatsoever so far as that was concerned. An oxygen tent was erected around her bed and doctors arrived immediately to examine her. Sara's admission to the Leeds General Infirmary was definitely the turning point in her life. I had been keeping a diary recording her condition and experiences for quite some time, and they show clearly that, whatever depths we had plumbed before, from this time onwards we were on the uphill climb.

Gradually, while Sara was a patient in the infirmary, I was able to tell the doctors there something of her history. It made a grim tale. I was able to substantiate the incredible number of attacks which she had suffered, not to mention the amazing catalogue of medical blunders which we had encountered, by referring to my 'Sara Diary'. Sara underwent every relevant test possible during her admission and not once did she show the slightest sign of distress, much less despair. I was more than welcome to stay with her as long as she needed me. Ward 56 was such a bright, happy, positive place to be; Sara and I knew that at last she was going to get better.

By the time she was discharged, emotionally speaking she was a different child. Gone were the moods and tantrums, and she was as exhilarated as I was by the improvement in her condition. Blood tests, which had not been carried out previously, showed that she could tolerate

a higher dose of Theophylin. Night-time coughing disappeared immediately. She was still to have the nebulised
solution of Intal four times a day and I was also given liquid
Ventolin for use in the nebuliser 'at the first sign of a
squeak', as the ward sister aptly put it.

# Chapter Ten

I stayed on at our house in Yorkshire with the children so that Sara could attend Outpatients and Physiotherapy on a regular basis; she still needed some physiotherapy to clear any remaining sticky mucus from her lungs. Her progress was excellent. At last the long-awaited moment arrived. Sara's next Outpatients appointment was set for three months' time, so I telephoned Steve and told him to expect us home for the summer. At long last it seemed that Sara's asthma was well and truly under control. There could not be any surprises left.

We all spent an idyllic summer together. It was just as if Sara had never been sick. We had frequently discussed the financial burden we endured by maintaining two homes and so regretfully we sold the house in Yorkshire. Things were going so well now for Sara that the sensible course seemed to be for us to live on the island where Steve's commitments to the business were inescapable, while I should fly to England every three months with Sara so that her condition could be monitored closely by the same team of doctors. We paid a 'flying' visit to our Yorkshire home and sold almost everything we had, putting only the most precious of our possessions into store until we had purchased a home on the island, at which time we would arrange for their transportation. We flew back to the apartment and I registered the children at school. We had most definitely 'burnt our boats', but financially, we had no alternative whatsoever.

The attack came without warning, during the second week of October. We called our GP who prescribed steroid medication in tablet form and told us that we would be very lucky to keep her out of hospital. The shock was brutal. My major concern was Sara's state of mind. Despite the ferocity of those many attacks and the appalling treatment which she had received in the island's hospital, Sara had, in a very mature way, put them all behind her and only considered how very well she had been looked after at the infirmary in Leeds, remembering the nurses who had played with her and the particular doctors she had favoured and looked upon as friends. Not a shadow of the nightmare she had endured on the island remained. To send her now to that 'prison camp' institution would be an appalling shock, and I feared it might have dreadful consequences. I determined then and there that if she was just lucky enough to avoid hospital admission this time, I would never put her at risk on the island again.

The consequence of this decision was clear: I must leave the island with the children for good, while Steve would eventually extricate himself as best he could from the business, upon which our very livelihood depended.

During the course of that long, melancholy night, we could see, to our immense relief, that Sara was beginning to recover. Our own 'home' nebuliser proved invaluable. We were able to administer the Ventolin every four hours during the night without once disturbing Sara.

The following day we set in motion the plans to take her home to England as soon as she was strong enough. The doctor called daily and, when he pronounced Sara fit to travel, she and I took the first available flight back to England. We were in something of a fix now, because we had nowhere to live. I arrived at my mother's with Sara, to pave the way for Steve and James, who were following on a later flight. It had proved impossible to book four seats together at such short notice. At this stage our plans were still rather vague, the main concern of everyone being simply to get Sara back into the care of the Leeds Royal Infirmary.

Sara was admitted immediately. X-rays showed once again that she was suffering from bronchopneumonia. I stayed with her in Ward 56, Steve returned to the island and James remained with my mother. Again Sara underwent a battery of tests. Doctors explained to me that they were repeating many tests which had been carried out previously at other hospitals, simply to satisfy themselves that they had been performed correctly. They reassured me that, despite Sara's continuing ill-health, it was unlikely that she was suffering from anything sinister. Her general appearance was still good, she looked sturdy and normal in every respect, but they emphasised the necessity to control her alarmingly unpredictable asthmatic condition.

Thankfully, the tests proved nothing other than the fact that her constant illness was solely attributable to her chronic asthma. No instantly recognisable 'triggers' were then, or ever have been, identified; the problem was how to prevent further attacks. It was imperative that Sara's lungs should have some respite from the incessant wheezing and asthma-induced infections which were an ever-present problem. The extremely high doses of steroids, which were undoubtedly 'life-saving' and essential during her worst attacks, although quite safe when used for isolated chronic attacks, were needed almost constantly in Sara's case because her attacks were almost always severe and came so very close together. This course of action could not be allowed to continue indefinitely. Obviously it was preferable to control the condition properly.

The doctors explained to me that drugs which would prove beneficial to Sara could only be found by a trial-and-error method. Medication which would prove invaluable in

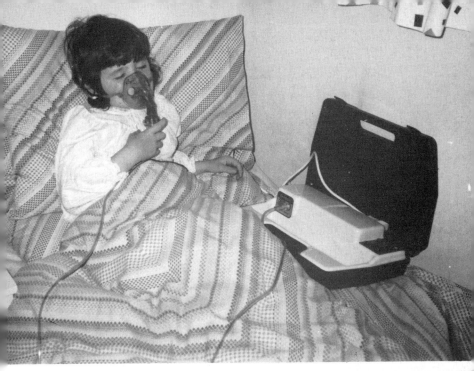

Sara using her nebuliser.

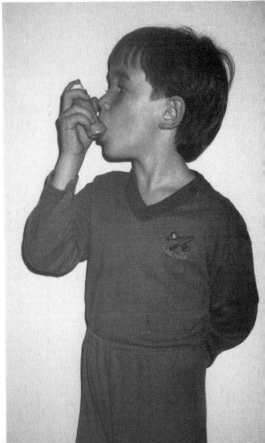

James using his pressurised
aerosol canister.

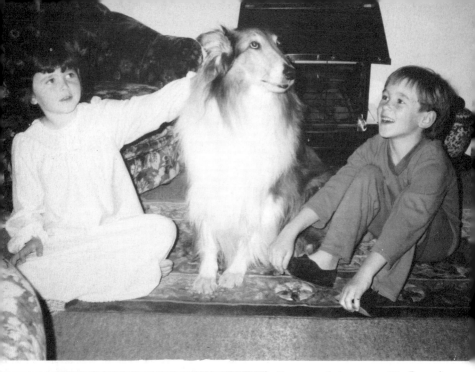

Sara and James with Bonnie - not all asthmatic children would be able to keep their pets like this.

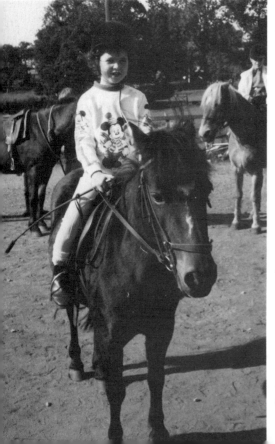

Sara with Tuesday. Riding gives her no problems.

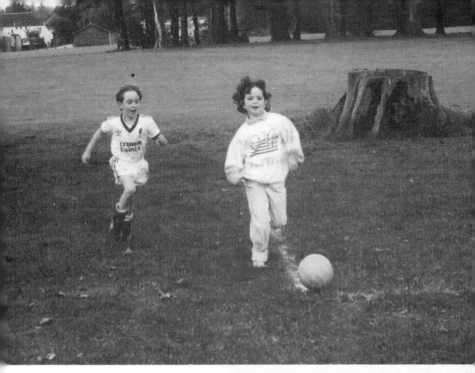

Games and energetic play are perfectly possible for asthmatic children.

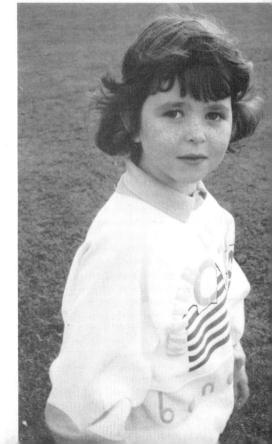

A happy, healthy little girl, who has learned to live with asthma.

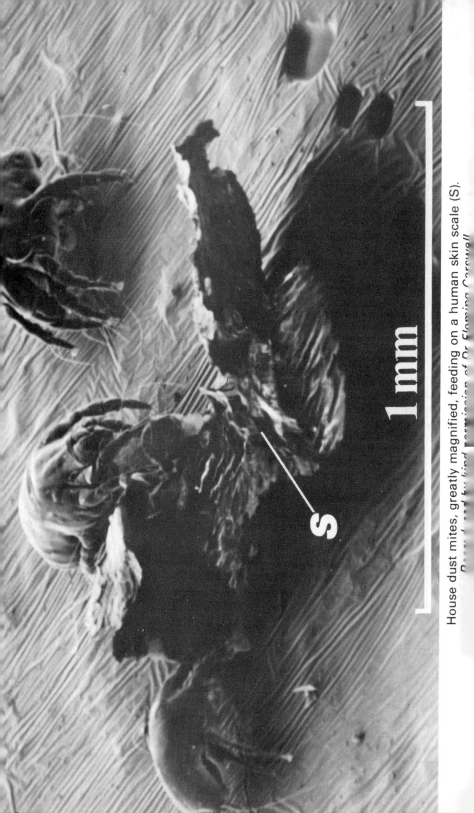

House dust mites, greatly magnified, feeding on a human skin scale (S).

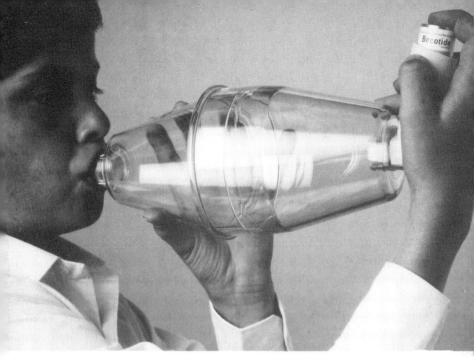

A Becotide pressurised aerosol being used in conjunction with a nebuhaler. *Photo: Allen and Hanburys Ltd.*

Child using a jet stream nebuliser. This is the hubble-bubble type that Sara found so difficult to master when she was very young. *Photo: Allen and Hanburys Ltd.*

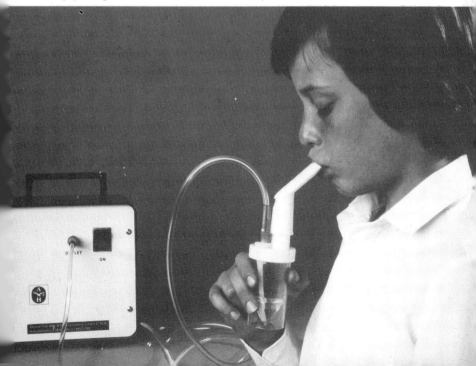

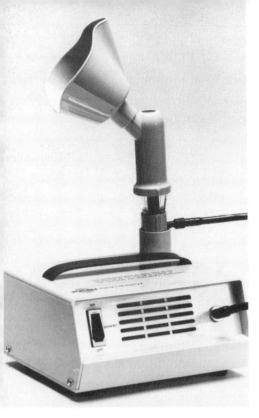

The Pari Inhalierboy, a
nebuliser of German
manufacture, driven by
compressed air. *Photo:
Clement Clarke International
Ltd.*

*Below:* The Pari Inhalierboy in
use. *Photo: Clement Clarke
International Ltd.*

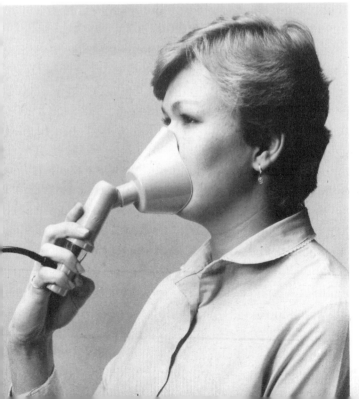

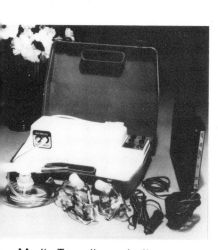

e Medix Traveller nebuliser
owing the jet nebuliser set, face-
ask and rechargeable battery pack
hich can be used with this
achine to give complete mobility.
oto: Medix Ltd.

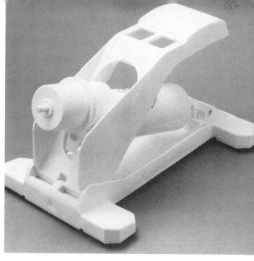

Foot or hand pump for the Easy Air
nebuliser which, again, offers
complete mobility and is very light
to carry around. *Photo: Cameron-
Price Medical Division Ltd.*

Child using a spinhaler. *Photo: Fisons Pharmaceuticals.*

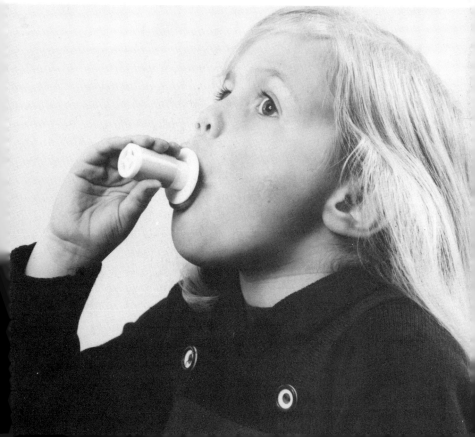

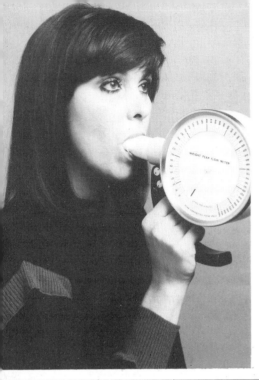

The Wright peak flow meter in use. This is the standard type suitable for adults. *Photo: Clement Clarke International Ltd.*

The low-range mini-Wright peak flow meter, ideal for children. *Photo: Clement Clarke International Ltd.*

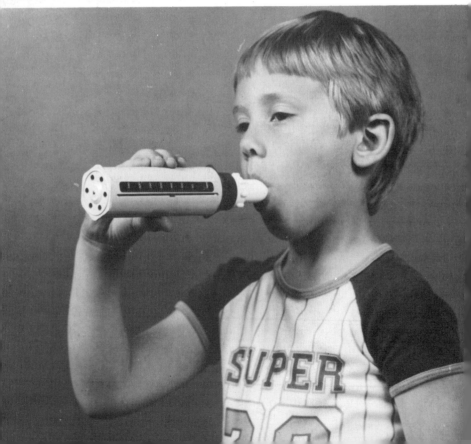

one child's case might not prove so effective in another's. They asked me not to be alarmed by the large amounts of drugs prescribed for Sara; they felt that the sort of 'blanket' treatment prescribed would provide the best hope of relief for her. The dose of Theophylin was raised slightly, and now both Ventolin and Becotide were to be inhaled four times a day using a rotahaler. Intal, so effective as a preventative in many cases, had proved ineffectual in Sara's case and so was dropped. When she was discharged we took home all of this, plus an antibiotic which she was to take for a short while, and also our supply of Ventolin solution with which I would be able to abort any mild attacks at home using the nebuliser. Quite an array!

I understood that I should not expect instant results; Becotide, for instance, would take a little while to become effective. The major benefit for Sara as far as I was concerned was that the doctors at the infirmary were determined to get to the bottom of her problem. There was no possibility that they would lose interest, or find it too much trouble to persist in seeking an answer, which I think had been partly to blame in the past. All the tension seemed to have been removed from me. There was a vigorous team of doctors who not only cared but intended to do something about Sara's miserable condition. If I had any queries or worries it was made quite clear to me that there would always be one of the team available to speak to me on the telephone, or I could take Sara along to the hospital at any time to a clinic or to the ward. The change this attitude wrought in our lives is beyond imagining. It simply removed all the fear, all the apprehension, and let Sara and me get on with living. 'Thank you' will never be enough: I could put no price on the product of their support.

Settling down at last to something approaching normality, I registered the children at the local school. All went smoothly until the onset of winter. Despite the fact that I had taken great care in advising the school's headmistress about Sara's condition, something which she could hardly dispute, having thanked me profusely for my detailed letter which was posted on the staff notice board, I discovered that Sara was being made to play outside at playtime in sometimes icy conditions. As soon as I learned what was happening, I visited the school to make known my concern. The headmistress was very pleasant, but determined. She informed me that if a child is well enough to go to school, she is well enough to play outside, surely a crass piece of misjudgement when applied to Sara. Secondly, when the sun shone it would 'do her good' to be outside, benefiting from the fresh air. To her first point, my reaction was amazement as I considered whether all the school's rules might be so inflexibly and insensitively applied. To her second point, I explained that it was not the sun which would do Sara good on a freezing-cold day, but the icy winds which would do her harm.

To underline my attitude and also to prove that I was not simply being difficult, I rang one of the doctors at the hospital, explaining what had happened and asking whether he would be good enough to send a letter outlining Sara's special needs with regard to her condition. The following letter arrived at our home by return of post:

Dear Sir/Madam,

Re: Sara Sutherland d.o.b. 6.5.79.

This young asthmatic child was recently on the ward with pneumonia. This has not cleared completely and at the moment it is inadvisable for her to be outside in extreme weather conditions as it may exacerbate her problem.

What a disgrace that a letter like this should be necessary.

To discuss the matter further with the headmistress was

irrelevant in any case. Sara's chest condition had already deteriorated. That woman could hardly have been surprised when, shortly afterwards, I removed both my children from her care.

If, for any reason, you are worried that your child's asthma is made worse at school, discuss the situation with your doctor who may be able to suggest a possible alternative within your catchment area. A letter from your doctor to the Schools Allocation Department of the relevant Education Authority, explaining the situation, should enable your child to move to a more suitable school, providing, of course, numbers permit.

Shortly after this incident, Sara suffered another attack. This was almost certainly caused by her recovery having been interrupted and her condition aggravated by exposure to the icy weather conditions. The difference now was that I was able simply to telephone the ward and warn them that we would be arriving. Sara received treatment within half-an-hour of the onset of the attack and, thankfully, it was aborted in its early stages. There is no doubt whatsoever in my mind that speed is of the essence when trying to avoid a serious attack. If I do not see an improvement within minutes of Sara finishing a nebulised dose of Ventolin, or if I notice that she is actually becoming more distressed even while she is inhaling the drug, I do not hesitate to take her straight to the hospital. On this last occasion Sara's recovery was swift. She had to attend Physiotherapy for some time as an outpatient, to ensure that her chest was completely free from mucus, and we ourselves also practised at home the methods used by the physiotherapist, as additional back-up. Her regular dose of the drug Becotide was increased and her other medications maintained at their previous levels.

The general opinion expressed by doctors is to favour sending asthmatic children back to school as soon as possible following an attack, for unless your child has had a particularly disturbed night and is obviously exhausted, or is still suffering from any residual infection caused by an attack and undergoing treatment for this, she must take every opportunity to live as normally as possible. It will not help her at all if you become apprehensive and over-protective. Asthmatic children should be receiving sufficient treatment from their doctors to enable them to attend school regularly. A little coughing or wheezing during the night is not a good enough reason to keep them at home. Sara, like most asthmatic children, is particularly liable to wheeze first thing in the morning, but this usually responds quite quickly to her medications, and I certainly would not keep her away from school because of this— providing of course that she sounds quite clear by the time we are ready to leave the house. When Sara has been in hospital with an attack, or is at home under the supervision of our GP, I always ask his advice as to when she should return to school. Occasionally, common sense dictates that she should not play outside or join in games, and most schools are only too willing to comply with these requests, providing of course you explain the situation clearly.

Make sure the school is aware of your child's condition; and I would not suggest simply having a chat about it—put the *facts* down in writing, they have a lot of other children to think about. A list of telephone numbers is essential, in case they are unable to contact you should your child have an attack which causes concern. So, leave the numbers of another relative or friend who could be called upon, of your GP and even the local hospital. Perhaps it may be possible to leave some spare medications with the school nurse or head teacher, thus enabling them to cope with a mild attack.

Make sure that the people who are likely to be the ones to help at your child's school know what to do if an attack occurs. It is important that they understand how to make your child as comfortable as possible until assistance, e.g. parent, friend, doctor, ambulance, arrives, or medicine takes effect. A well-intentioned person might try to make the child lie down.

But if they know the best way to treat a child during an asthma attack, they themselves will be less likely to panic, which would only alarm the child and exacerbate the attack. A simple check-list could be written underneath your child's medicine timetable and kept at the school. You will know what helps your own child better than anyone, but something along these lines would be helpful: Loosen top clothing—school tie, top buttons, etc. Sit the child up, well supported by pillows, cushions, etc. (Some children like to lean forward, although Sara never did.) An older child might prefer to stand and lean over, supporting herself against the back of a stable chair. The most important thing to remember is that someone stays with her until either the attack subsides or help arrives. She should *not* be left alone.

Undoubtedly, children pick up more infections when they begin to go to school, and these infections may well precipitate asthma attacks. There is really no way round this; your child must go to school, but it does pay to be prepared. There are a few special schools for those children who suffer from particularly acute asthma. These are boarding schools where the children are shown how to live with their asthma. They learn that they *can* play games, attend lessons regularly and live a full, active life. Some children benefit enormously from this sort of protective environment. Your doctor would be the best person to advise you about the suitability of this particular option, as the individual needs of each child differ so greatly.

Sara is still extremely susceptible to chest infections and we never become careless or complacent about either her medications or her condition. I am on 'red alert' all the time and would notice the slightest change in her health immediately. Our stock of pills and potions never becomes low and I have spare 'puffers' squirrelled away in case we lose one. Sara may need some form of medication to hand indefinitely, but at the moment we have reached the happy stage where she is gradually being 'weaned off' some of the drugs. So far, so good, but it is a long, cautious programme, requiring constant monitoring by her doctors and taking place over many months. I can still remember the early days of her treatment. How confusing it all seemed. It is terribly hard to be objective and receptive to information when you are numb with shock after receiving the doctor's diagnosis. If the doctor goes too fast and you do not take it all in first time round, do not be embarrassed about asking him to repeat everything slowly, while you make a few notes. Then, when you return home, you can write out your own timetable and label the various drugs so that you are absolutely confident about when and how they are to be used.

Nothing makes me happier then being able to tell you that Sara is now able to lead a completely normal life—and for an asthmatic whose condition is successfully controlled, that is exactly how it should be. Those seemingly endless days and nights of ever-present tension and apprehension are past, month upon month of waiting for 'the cough', history.

I encountered further proof of this successful control a short time ago. Sara executed a flamboyant somersault over the handlebars of her new bicycle. She was admitted to hospital, suffering from concussion. While delirious, she interspersed her ramblings with frantic, hysterical shrieks which continued for several exhausting hours. I felt sure that her wild behaviour must surely precipitate a serious attack . . . nothing!

I could be hypercritical and allow that the control of Sara's asthma can never eradicate every last clue to her condition. A balance which is both effective and safe must be reached when such a long-term programme of medications is implemented. If we had had no experience whatsoever of asthma and were to hear Sara breathing at certain times, we might comment that 'her chest sounds a bit wheezy', or, 'she has some catarrh on her chest'. A nip in the air, slight infection, excitement, etc., all the old adversaries, still provoke Sara's airways into reacting in a typical, although thankfully now extremely mild, asthmatic pattern.

I refer to this pattern as an example of the predominant state of Sara's health. However, following eighteen months of freedom from the now readily identifiable wheezing attacks, Sara has been admitted to hospital three times over the recent winter months with pneumonia and persistent partial collapse of one of her lungs. These conditions are solely attributable to her asthma.

There is no indication from her doctors at present that they intend to increase the dosage of her drugs, but these events demonstrate the delicate balance upon which control of the disease depends, and underlines more emphatically than anything else I can tell you, the dangers of complacency and the truly desperate need for a cure.

Illness, and our comparisons of those symptoms associated with a particular disease are all a matter of degree. For us, considering how chronically and continuously sick Sara has been, she is now 'better'. However, because that disparity still persists when comparing Sara with her non-asthmatic friends, and depressing set-backs still occur from time to time, I continue to hope that one day she will be cured and rid of her asthma forever.

When I first began to write this book, I could not be sure that Sara's condition would ever improve to any worthwhile degree—and, to be honest, I was not very optimistic. If you could see her now, you would agree that it is impossible to tell that she has ever been so terribly ill, or that so many drugs are still very much a part of her everyday routine.

Far from suffering any adverse reactions to some of the appalling things which have happened to her, she is mature, resourceful and courageous. Recently, brushing off our concern after a fall at her first gymkhana, she remounted her pony and continued the competition, winning sufficient points to clinch the championship. Once she was assured that the trophy was safely hers, I drove us both to hospital, where an X-ray showed that she had cracked her elbow. To Sara, after all her other tribulations, the pain which this must have caused was as inconsequential as a pinprick might have been to the rest of us.

I would not even try to put a number to those occasions when I thought Sara would never be well, and I could not possibly have imagined that the day would come when I would be able to write about her improvement with such confidence. But, that day came for us, and I am sure it will for you, too, so long as you do not give up.

# PART II

## FACTS AND QUESTIONS

Sara's story illustrates the experiences of only one child and her family, but I hope that readers will have found similarities with the problems they have had to face, and that our mistakes will help them avoid the same pitfalls. There are, however, practical steps that we can all take to smooth the path for our children, and in this part of the book I shall attempt to raise—and answer—the numerous questions that parents of an asthmatic child will want to ask. Many of these points could not have been answered to my complete satisfaction without the constant support and encouragement which I have received from the Asthma Society and Friends of the Asthma Research Council.

First of all, I should like to look at the most corrosive emotion that can ever strike parents of asthmatic children.

## Guilt

One of the worst things I have had to come to terms with—and this, I suspect, is an experience common to most parents of asthmatic children—has been my own feeling of guilt. The sick feeling of apprehension I feel whenever *I* wake up with a sore throat, or James or Steve have some minor infection, has never left me. A small inconvenience for us can prove to be a major problem for Sara. Protected as she is by so many medications, more often than not a serious attack is avoided, even if she does contract our infection, but very occasionally she succumbs to an acute asthma attack and this for me, as, I am sure, for every other parent of an asthmatic child, seems to happen when I am most confident and complacent, secure in the illusion that . . . it will never happen again.

In retrospect, I know that I could have done things better, and acted more quickly to help Sara in the early days of her illness, if only I, as a member of the general public, had been better informed about asthma. But even when I became better informed, I still worried in case I was, however unwittingly, aggravating Sara's condition. Was I expecting too much of her? Pushing her too hard to do well at school? I can remember going hot and cold with concern when people asked me questions about Sara when they learned that she was asthmatic. I was asked whether she was nervous, highly strung, unusually emotional, as if all I must do was keep her calm and she would be well, whereas, to be honest, when unaffected by a wheezing attack she seemed to be perfectly calm already. Yet still the niggling doubt persisted: Had I missed something that other people could see and I could not? Was I doing something wrong which had precipitated her asthmatic condition? Now at last, to these questions I can answer most emphatically, no. As far as I can judge by comparing Sara to her peers, and indeed to James, she appears to be completely normal—both in behaviour and misbehaviour!

Some investigations have in fact been carried out to try to identify an 'asthmatic personality', but as yet, no one has been able to prove that such a thing exists. I realise now that all my early worries were totally unfounded; Sara's asthma improved just as soon as the doctors identified the most effective course of treatment for her.

## Problem Thunderstorm
Recent research by two specialists at an East Birmingham hospital, dispelled some of the worries of other asthmatics and their parents.

A severe thunderstorm on 6th and 7th July, 1983,

heralded the arrival of an unusual number of asthma patients requiring emergency treatment at the hospital. Many thought that the cause of their attack was 'nerves', a result, they assumed, of having been frightened by the storm. Research suggested that thunderstorms themselves can trigger serious attacks by releasing microscopic fungal spores into the air. These are so light that they are not washed out of the atmosphere by rain, and so can cause an allergic reaction when they are breathed in. Another reason put forward to explain deterioration in asthma during thunderstorms, is that the number of positive ions in the air increases at these times.

When the doctors analysed the outbreak in Birmingham, they found that, for most of June and July, eight Birmingham hospitals treated between two and twenty asthma patients a day—on July 6th, it leaped to thirty-six cases, and on July 7th, to a record seventy. Another thirteen hospitals in the West Midlands reported that asthma cases had tripled during the storm.

Doctors in Nottingham have also confirmed that recent storms in their area have had a similar effect. One doctor commented: 'Clearly more research is needed into the effect of thunderstorms on asthma patients.'

Whether or not thunderstorms prove in themselves to have relevance where increased numbers of acute attacks are noted in hospitals, I find interesting the fact that on practically every occasion Sara has been admitted to hospital in a chronic condition, whatever the weather or season, it has been mentioned by either doctor or nurse that there has been an unusually large number of asthmatics admitted that same day or thereabouts. I can see for myself on Ward 56 at Leeds General Infirmary, how many of the 'old gang' inevitably arrive to take up their beds in the 'asthma bay'. Whether this coincides with children returning to school after the holidays and so picking up infections, or whether climatic conditions, seasonal changes, etc., play a part remains to be proved. But it is certainly interesting and surely relevant to note that, in some instances at least, asthma, like infectious diseases, can occur in waves.

## Explanations

Your child will probably come to terms with her asthma more quickly if you take the time to explain to her exactly what is going on. What is the point of glossing over her condition, when much of the responsibility for treatment must ultimately fall into the child's own hands? When she understands that as many as one in ten other children suffer from asthma symptoms, too, she will realise that there is nothing odd or embarrassing about her condition.

As soon as possible, teach your child what to do if she begins to feel unwell, and help her to recognise those situations which are liable to trigger an attack, so that she can either prepare for them, e.g. by remembering to take her medications before games; or, avoid them, e.g. particular allergens.

There is no reason why even quite a young child should not be allowed to go to, say, a birthday party—so long as the hosts know where to contact you if necessary; before she could remember it for herself, Sara always had our telephone number written in her shoes. If food allergies are a problem, there is not a mum alive who will object to your child taking a packed party snack with her, and, in my experience, when Sara was on an exclusion diet, it was *her* food which proved to be the big attraction, because it was different. So, although it was probably the one occasion when she consumed her regulation carrot candies with real relish, she suffered no embarrassment and certainly missed none of the fun.

To guard against other small children at school playing with, breaking, losing or even using your child's inhaler, it will be necessary to let a member of staff keep it safe for you, but an older child will probably want to keep it with her and use her own discretion as to when to use it, e.g. it may become necessary in the middle of sports. Older children may also like to keep a timetable or chart of their medications for themselves—perhaps in a handy notebook— and tick off the appropriate treatment as it is used. You might, however, feel happier if your child's use of her medicine is monitored by a member of staff, for although children will not become addicted to their asthma medications, they may build up a certain emotional dependency on the drug and so unwittingly overdose themselves. It is also possible that they might forget how many times they have used their inhaler if this use becomes too casual.

Especially with younger children, I think it is important for their teacher to find a good moment to talk to the class in simple terms about asthma—particularly the fact that it is not catching! Children can be very cruel when they do not understand, but very supportive once their curiosity has been satisfied.

## Heredity and Asthma

I have heard it said that asthmatic children whose parents or close relatives have asthma are less likely to improve as they grow older than other asthmatic children; this remains unproven and certainly, if you have severe asthma yourself and your child is also asthmatic, it will not automatically follow that he or she will suffer from exactly the same degree of asthma as you. There is evidence that heredity plays a part in the incidence of asthma, but the severity of the condition has not been found to run consistently through a family.

This fact was clearly demonstrated in my own family when we discovered that James also suffered from asthma, although his was in a very mild form. His condition was easily identified in the light of our previous experience with Sara, and so brought under control almost before he realised that there was anything wrong. James has exercise-induced asthma (see p. 127), which means that he becomes short of breath very quickly when playing games, running, etc. Occasionally he, too, experiences the night-time cough. This was found to be totally unaffected by treatment with the usual children's cough remedies, but responded quickly to asthma medications; in his case, the bronchodilator, Ventolin, used in a rotahaler.

The doctor also tested him with a 'peak flow meter', to confirm her diagnosis. This is a simple device into which the child is required to blow as hard as he can, to measure the speed with which he is able to force the air out of his lungs. When the airways are tight, the rate at which the air can be forced out drops, so this method provides the doctor with a simple way of assessing the constriction in the airways. The child can then be tested again after he has used a bronchodilator, or other treatment at the doctor's discretion; in this way his response to various medications can be determined. Normal values vary according to the age, sex, musculature and body-build of each individual, but a simple chart called a 'nomogram', showing the normal range, is available from Clement Clarke International Ltd., 15 Wigmore Street, London W1H 9LA.

### Games

James uses his 'puffer' immediately before games and again during exercise if he becomes breathless, wheezy, or coughs at all. There is no reason why asthmatic children should not participate in games so long as they have the appropriate medications which allow them to take part without experiencing any discomfort.

My children excel at swimming and this is one of the best exercises of all for an asthmatic. Apart from the obvious benefits of exercising and strengthening the whole body, the air immediately above a heated pool is warm and humid and these conditions are less likely to produce wheezing.

Endurance sports are perhaps more difficult for the

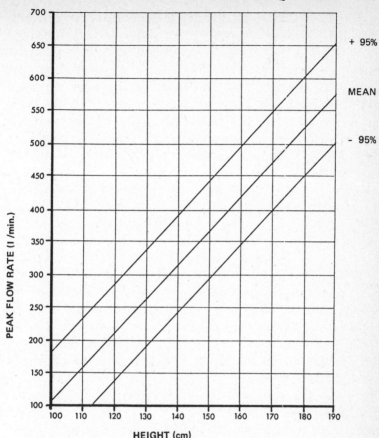

This nomogram results from tests carried out by Dr. S. Godfrey and his colleagues on a sample of 382 normal boys and girls aged 5 to 18 years. Each child blew 5 times into a standard Wright Peak Flow Meter and the highest reading was accepted in each case. All measurements were completed within a 6-week period. The outer lines of the graph indicated that the results of 95% of the children fell within these boundaries.

(Redrawn from original data of Godfrey et al Brit.J.Dis.Chest, *64*, 15 (1970). Reproduced by kind permission of Clement Clarke International Ltd.)

asthmatic but *not* impossible—Steve Ovett proved this point rather conclusively!

## Pets

The general rule of thumb is: do not introduce any new furry or feathered pets into the household. Even if your child does not appear to be allergic to your present pet, she may well develop an allergy to a new one over a period of time, thus adding to her problems. If you already have a pet in the home and your child suffers from year-round asthma, you do have to consider the possibility that your pet could be causing an allergic reaction. Some clues to watch out for when you are trying to discover whether or not your child is allergic to animals are given in the section *Asthma and Allergy*.

If your child is desperate to try something like horse riding, where the contact with the animal is outside the home, why not let her try? You will soon find out how she fares, and you will not be left with an unwanted pet if she does become wheezy and decide not to continue. I took Sara along to the stables with me a couple of times to see what would happen; she now goes riding regularly. Caution and common sense will dictate what you do and do not allow your child to do.

Now I have a confession to make: we have a dog, a large, hairy collie. 'Ah!' you shriek in righteous indignation, 'how could she?' We had Bonnie before Sara was born. I realise that allergies can develop over a period of time, so the fact that Sara lived with a dog in the house for some twenty months without suffering an allergic reaction is not relevant. However, Sara's condition deteriorated during the period of time when Bonnie was already back in England for her six months quarantine period, and the dog was back home with us when Sara's condition was eventually controlled successfully. Proximity to Bonnie, or indeed any other animal, seems to have not the slightest effect on Sara's health. I realise that Sara is one of the lucky ones, being able to keep her beloved pet, and mention this just in case some other child might also be able to keep her animal. Again, common sense and the advice of your doctor are the yardsticks to use when considering whether it is advisable to keep an existing pet. I am sure that, if I had known about Sara's asthma before having a dog, I would not have bought one for her, as it would have been impossible to judge whether she might develop an allergy to it over a period of time.

Regrettably, it remains at the back of my mind that, should Sara ever develop an allergy at some time in the future, either to Bonnie or some other animal, we, too, would have to review our stance regarding her contact with them.

## Breath Control and Yoga

Anything which promotes calm, controlled breathing is obviously going to help an asthmatic. Learning to play a wind instrument is just one way in which an older child might learn to develop this sort of control. Another excellent activity is yoga. Studies have been completed recently on the beneficial effects of yoga exercises on asthma patients. Yoga has long been recognised as having a calming as well as fitness-promoting effect, and it makes perfect sense to consider this sort of exercise very seriously. The study, which was published in the *British Medical Journal*, compared two similar groups of asthmatics. The patients in one group practised yoga regularly and found that they had fewer attacks and so required fewer drugs than those in the other group. Better breath control, however achieved, must benefit your child to some degree, although is unlikely to provide the complete answer.

## Relaxation Exercises

I practised relaxation and breathing exercises with Sara,

which I had learnt during my years at music college, as part of my training to become an opera singer. Quite simply, we started with a deep breath in through the nose for a count of three; held for three; exhaled slowly through the mouth, also for a count of three. The shoulders must not be allowed to move at all as you practise this exercise. To ensure that your child is breathing deeply enough, place her hands, with fingertips touching, across her diaphragm, thumbs hooked around her sides. When she breathes in correctly, the fingertips should move apart. This exercise can be repeated as frequently as you wish.

Another exercise that we do requires gentle, controlled movements of the upper body while Sara is breathing deeply and regularly, in through the nose and out through the mouth. She aims to achieve a harmonious rhythm between her movements and her breathing. She starts by rolling her head gently round in a clockwise circle. Her mouth is allowed to fall open as her head goes back to avoid any strain on the throat or neck. The head must not drop forward suddenly, indeed there must be no sudden jerks at all; just a smooth, steady movement, breathing in through the nose as the head circles backwards, and out again through the mouth as the head moves slowly forwards and down to rest on her chest again. Sara then repeats the exercise in an anti-clockwise direction, using the same breathing pattern as before.

Sara's favourite exercise is when she pretends to be a rag doll. She relaxes forwards from the waist and bounces gently, then peels back gradually into an upright position, breathing steadily all the while.

There is no doubt in my mind that these exercises help to promote relaxation and certainly take a child's mind off her asthma, but from our own experience I would not suggest that exercise alone will dramatically alter your child's condition.

## What about the Heart and Lungs?

One of the most frightening aspects of Sara's severe asthma attacks has been the dramatic increase in her pulse rate. During the worst occasions it would rise dramatically and remain high for long periods of time. This frantic pumping of her heart, combined with the all-too obvious demands placed upon her overworked lungs, led me to wonder whether she might suffer some permanent damage. The reassurances given to me at the time have thankfully proved accurate. A child's heart is more than able to cope with even the most severe attack, and her lungs are similarly resilient. Recent examinations show Sara's heart and lungs to be as normal and healthy as those of a non-asthmatic child.

## Air Travel

Holidays involving air travel do not have to be avoided. There is a drop in the level of oxygen present in the aircraft cabin at high altitudes, and although this has never caused Sara any discomfort, at one time during long flights she would have to use her nebuliser on the aeroplane to take her medicine (Intal) at the usual time. As I mentioned before, the foot pump nebuliser adapts itself readily to most situations, being light to carry, self-contained and incidentally much cheaper to buy than the electric model. Remember also that oxygen is readily available on an aircraft should it be necessary.

## Clothing

As far as clothing is concerned, apart from normal concern to ensure that your child is warm enough, does not stay in wet clothes too long, or puts damp clothes on, there is no evidence to show that bundling up her chest with layers of woolly vests will help her asthma at all. However, in very cold or windy weather, I have found that a scarf over Sara's mouth is a great help in preventing her from breathing asthma-provoking dust or icy air directly into her lungs.

## The Asthma Attack

Is there really anything worse? For the asthmatic, however young or old, it feels as if she is choking, as if huge weights are pressing down relentlessly on her chest. There can be nothing more frightening than being unable to breathe—and it is hardly less so for the parent who must stand and watch.

When your child is frightened it makes her asthma worse. Think how breathless you get when you have a sudden shock. If you allow your own alarm to show you are only going to make matters much worse. I know only too well how difficult it is, but you really must call on all your reserves of strength and remain calm, no matter what. Something that will help is to make certain that you are always prepared for an attack. You do not want to be rushing around the house in a state of panic, looking for medicine, telephone numbers, pieces of nebuliser or whatever. Keep everything together in one place close at hand, even when you are out, if your child's asthma is particularly unpredictable. Obviously, if there are other people about, they can do the running about for you while you stay and comfort the child; otherwise, organise yourself with the minimum of fuss. First, ensure that the child is reassured and placed in the most comfortable position for her (see p. 101). Remember, she is looking to you for help; you must be positive and take control. A soothing, confident attitude will help to eliminate anxiety, but at the same time remain vigilant for the slightest sign of deterioration.

If an attack does not respond within a reasonable period of time to treatment with a bronchodilator such as Ventolin or whatever your doctor has prescribed (by 'reasonable period of time' I mean at most half-an-hour, or *less* if there are obvious signs of deterioration), call the doctor. If the doctor is not *immediately* available, go straight to your nearest Casualty Department. Even before Sara was permitted to go straight to the ward at the infirmary as a known asthmatic, during a severe attack she has always been given priority in Casualty in this country. Never feel that an asthma attack is not sufficient reason to go to Casualty; it is.

A mild attack may respond well to treatment given at home. Stay with your child, see her through it, but do not 'harp' on it. Distract her if possible with a story, or even a television programme, but nothing helps more than a calm, loving atmosphere. Sara positively 'feeds' off me when she is distressed. Her eyes lock onto mine and the slightest sign of fear or apprehension on my part would be communicated to her instantly. It goes without saying, I am sure, that it is essential to ensure that a sufficient quantity of your child's particular medication is always readily available. It is all too easy to run short. Imagine how much more alarmed your child will become if her medicine has run out.

Never cease or reduce medications without the express direction of your doctor. Once, beset with concern regarding the vast quantity of drugs which Sara was taking, I foolishly decided to omit her night-time capsule of Theophylin, to 'see what happens'—she coughed all night. I never made that mistake again. On a subsequent occasion, I simply forgot to give her the capsule. The result was the same: the unpleasant night-time cough returned.

It is imperative to follow the instructions of your doctor meticulously with regard to all the prescribed medications. Moreover, if you find that your child needs to use her inhaler more frequently, or if it is no longer effective, you must contact your doctor immediately, as the treatment may need adjusting.

Once an attack has subsided and the doctor pronounces your child's chest 'free from wheeze' or, 'no longer tight', the child may still be left with an unpleasant wet-sounding, chesty cough. I find with Sara that this cough may last for a week or slightly longer, as it takes quite some time for the excess mucus produced during an attack to be dispersed, by coughing it up and natural absorption into the body. Providing she does not develop a temperature, denoting an infection, I realise that this cough is a normal if disagreeable sequel to an acute attack.

## Don't Settle for Second Best

Never give up the search for a doctor who is sympathetic to your problem. You would be surprised to find just how accessible the really good doctors can be. Even specialists are not as elusive as you might suppose. In our experience, the doctors who possess the ability and the desire to help will always find time to see a sick child. Sadly, at the present time, an actual cure simply does not exist for asthma. What you should be looking for is successful long-term management of the illness, to control and suppress the unpleasant symptoms. A cavalier, dismissive attitude is just not good enough when it comes both to finding this solution and to handling the close monitoring which will be necessary for the proper control of your child's condition.

I have no professional dignity upon which to stand, and if, during the course of Sara's story, I appear to have been dilatory in my response to her early problems, it is because I was. I made the biggest blunders of anyone, because I did not understand what asthma was, and I simply was not forceful enough on Sara's behalf. If our experiences can enable even one person to act more positively, then relating Sara's story exactly as it happened has been more than worthwhile.

My feelings towards the medical profession are still somewhat ambivalent. On the one hand, we have encountered some wonderful doctors, imbued with genuine concern for their patients. To a few others I would say, intellect is not an automatic passport to respect. Reflect on the possibility that a patient or attendant relative may be equally well qualified in his or her own particular field, although largely ignorant of medical matters and their attendant 'jargon'. Certain words and phrases, although commonplace among medical folk, may be obscure generally. Do not patronise us 'laypeople'; do not shut us out. You are not mechanics dealing with inanimate objects! We have a right to know.

Consider further that a child's parents may be suffering from considerable shock when informed that their child is an asthmatic, and so not thinking clearly. It is essential that doctors take the time and trouble to explain thoroughly, at the earliest time following diagnosis, both the consequences and implications of asthma—also carefully defining the purpose of each drug so that the likelihood of complacency regarding their necessity is eradicated completely. There must always be room in the medical world for sensitivity, most especially when dealing with children. I have been told that doctors require a minimum IQ of 125 before they are able to commence their rigorous training. Jolly good for them—but, might it not also be a good idea, once their doctorate is achieved, if they embark upon a good course in public relations?

Neither must you allow your child to be treated as if she always brings on her asthma attacks herself, solely as a means of manipulating a situation to her advantage, e.g. missing school, avoiding a scolding, etc. Doctors agree that, in some instances it is possible for an asthmatic to bring on an attack—but the asthmatic condition *must* be present to start with. Tension and tempers may well aggravate the problem, but these are not the root cause of asthma. Perhaps we have avoided this situation with Sara because she knows we would not succumb. If she has a tantrum I leave her to it and get on with something else. Emotional dramatics usually need the stimulus of an audience.

The most important thing to remember, once you have done everything in your power to ensure that your child's asthma is as well controlled as it possibly can be, is to get on with your own life. Do not let asthma become the hub of your family's existence around which everything else is expected to revolve. It is only *one* problem—and there are bound to be plenty more in the years to come.

## Asthma and Allergy

Allergy: An abnormal sensitivity to a specific substance (such as food, pollen, dust, etc.) or condition (heat, cold, damp, wind, etc.) which in similar amounts is harmless to most people.

The major catch is the fact that an allergy can develop over several years, and when it finally manifests itself it remains undetected, because the sufferer mistakenly thinks that as he has always been immune to something, he always will be immune to it . . . wrong!

The most common causes of allergic asthma are pollen, house dust, house dust mite, animal skin, fur, saliva, feathers, fine dust carried on the wind, fumes, mould spores, drugs, food, trees—the list could go on and on; there are so many potentially provocative substances around us. One of the very worst is cigarette smoke; never smoke near an asthmatic, and by fumes I refer not only to obvious strong odours, but also to perfumes, paints, cleaning agents and the smell from new carpets, etc.

It is almost impossible to avoid allergens such as pollen or mould spores. They are microscopic and can be carried for miles in the air. Only the rain can impede their progress, and obviously, when weather conditions are still and sunny they are not gathered up and launched on their travels in quite such vast quantities.

Staying indoors with the windows shut, even using air filtration units and ionisers to 'cleanse' the air, would seem pointless, not to mention irksome; firstly, because it surely would not be possible to remain indoors for the whole of the summer to avoid the worst of the pollen season, not forgetting that mould spores are a year-round hazard; and secondly, even were you to use a filtration unit or ioniser, it would need to be on twenty-four hours a day to be even remotely effective—and what happens when you leave the room?

Various machines are available in the shops, marketed as creating a beneficial atmosphere for the asthmatic's bedroom. Tread warily; these may be expensive and are scientifically unproven. Even the most sophisticated air conditioner would not cope satisfactorily with every particle of dust or pollen. Think how much pollen or dust might be brought into a room unwittingly on shoes or clothing. If you really want to try this sort of thing, do not buy, but borrow a machine and draw your own conclusions. If the asthmatic feels reassured and happier with such a machine in the room, her symptoms might well subside—and that in itself may make the purchase worthwhile.

Allergy to animals is unfortunately more common among children than adults, with cats and birds heading the list of likely allergy provokers. You will know if your child is allergic to, or has developed an allergy to, an animal if, shortly after coming into contact with it, she has an attack of coughing or wheezing; sometimes this may be combined with sneezing, streaming eyes and runny noses. Dogs, guinea pigs, hamsters, gerbils, rabbits, mice, in fact any furry creature you can think of, may cause an allergic reaction. Caged birds are another of the worst offenders.

Sometimes horses provoke asthma symptoms; and horsehair, whether on your clothing or in the stuffing of your furniture, is a potential allergen. Some 'pony mad' children do overcome this problem by using a bronchodilator before coming into contact with horses. It is up to the individual to gauge whether her symptoms can be controlled sufficiently by this method, so that she can enjoy her riding. *Whenever possible* it is quite right that an asthmatic child should want to do all the things which a non-asthmatic child is able to do.

If children are allergic to a pet in the home, you have a problem. Getting rid of an animal which your child is attached to is going to upset her dreadfully, and this in itself will probably make her asthma worse. Even if you do remove her pet, it is extremely unlikely that her asthma symptoms will disappear altogether, since they are almost certainly due to a number of other reasons as well.

Perhaps the pet could live outside? This would reduce the skin, hair and saliva debris inside the home. If not, perhaps a sympathetic friend or relative might be prepared to keep the animal for a few weeks; then you will be able to see if there really is a worthwhile improvement in your child's condition.

Failing this, you really do not have much option but to try to find some 'safe' alternative pets to interest your child. There are some beautiful fish available, which could be built up into an interesting and decorative collection, both tropical varieties and pond fish. Koi, in particular, can be encouraged and trained, by using a pond-side bell, to come when you are ready to feed them, and will eventually take the food from your fingers. I had thought that perhaps a tortoise or even terrapins might make interesting pets until I contacted the Aquarium Department of Leeds University to enquire about their suitability. I am afraid that the opinions expressed were not in favour of keeping these types of creatures as pets. I was told that tortoises are rarely kept properly and as a consequence die in huge numbers during the winter, thus seriously depleting the ranks of this declining species. As for terrapins, they should never be removed from their natural habitat. Both were said to be imported from 'questionable' sources in many instances, with the very real possibility that they might carry disease. I am only sorry I cannot offer any other worthwhile alternatives to those asthmatic pet lovers who cannot tolerate fur and feathers.

Even if your own home is pet-free, the child who is

allergic to animals may still have an attack when visiting other people's homes, or there may be pets kept at school. Older children will probably overcome this problem quite simply, by avoiding unnecessary contact with the animal and by using her bronchodilator whenever necessary. But do make certain for the young child, particularly in those situations where you will not be there to look out for her, for example at school, that she is not made to sit in a classroom where a school pet such as a rabbit is kept. Keep the school fully informed *in writing* (keep a copy), perhaps backed up by a letter from your doctor, and do not forget to 'up-date' the school whenever necessary regarding your child's condition.

It is said that male animals cause more problems than females, and short-haired dogs are more provocative than long-haired breeds. The same rule applies to cats. Siamese and Burmese cause more problems than their long-haired cousins. Whilst hair and skin scurf are allergy provokers, the dried saliva of cats also causes problems. As cat lovers will know, these animals devote a great deal of their time to grooming, which of course involves much fur-licking.

We all know what household dust looks like and have a pretty good idea what goes into its making. The most provocative and unpleasant component of all is the house dust mite. Unless you are lucky enough to live in the high, dry altitudes of the Alps—and I believe they are fairly scarce in the Polar regions!—you are going to house the mite in your home, despite all your most strenuous efforts to eliminate the creature.

The mite likes fairly warm, humid conditions and thrives particularly on mattresses, where there are plenty of human skin scales for it to feed on. Mites are almost invisible to the naked eye, and the only way you can try and protect an allergic child from them is to obtain a plastic mattress cover (free) for her bed—and any other bed in the room—from your doctor or from the hospital. Wipe this down every day. Change bedding regularly. Substitute synthetic-filled pillows and duvets for mite-harbouring feather, and, remembering how little chance of survival the mite has in the polar regions, if you have a freezer big enough, it is not as ridiculous as it might sound to wrap up your child's synthetic-filled duvet and pillows in a large plastic dustbin bag, perhaps once a week, and leave them in the freezer for a day—not forgetting to thaw them out in good time for bed, of course! Eliminate woolly blankets where possible. Damp-dust the room every day. Remove the carpet and replace it with washable floor covering. Discard soft toys, unless you are going to wash them all daily; perhaps keep one favourite, providing it is washable. What about the curtains? A spongeable blind might be better. All of this *may* help but, regrettably, some children show no improvement at all—so do not drive yourself mad. *You* may feel reassured, however, knowing that you have taken every conceivable precaution for your child, to help protect her during that long and most vulnerable time when she is asleep.

Do not vacuum, dust, make the beds, or do any other household activity which is likely to raise dust, while the asthmatic child is around and, of course, try to stop her from putting her face near the carpet or from burrowing into upholstered furniture.

Unfortunately, allergies which provoke asthma are not restricted to the things we breathe in; some foods may provoke a reaction. Certain medicines—aspirin, for instance —may trigger symptoms; and watch out for simple remedies, bought over the counter at the chemist, which are *loaded* with artificial colouring. Colorants and chemicals are like *dynamite* to an asthmatic child with food allergies. Another point to watch is the high sugar content in syrup-type medications. This can cause tooth decay and so it is important to ensure that your child cleans her teeth *after* taking the medicine.

If you are able to identify specific allergies in your asthmatic child, at least you can try to help her to avoid them, or take precautionary measures to ensure that there will be no reaction by, a) using a regular preventative treatment prescribed by your doctor to reduce the sensitivity of the child's airways, and b) using an inhaled bronchodilator before she comes into contact with a known 'trigger'.

There are a few special clinics where older children may be able to obtain desensitising injections. These will not cure their asthma, but might help a few of the children plagued by allergies to mites or pollen. However, because these injections are most likely to succeed the higher the dose and the longer period of time taken for the course, the inconvenience factor is high and there may be undesirable reactions. Not to put it too bluntly, they do not always work.

By the age of about seven children have built up some resistance to the sort of everyday infections which may provoke their asthma symptoms, and it is always worth looking at allergies as a most likely cause of trouble if their asthma symptoms persist beyond this age.

**Exercise Asthma**
Relatively simple to recognise, exercise asthma sets in shortly after any exertion which might be expected to leave a non-asthmatic person breathless. Whereas a non-asthmatic person gradually begins to get her breath back after a bout of exercise, an asthmatic finds that, although she may have been only a little short of breath during exercise, it is when she stops that her breathing becomes more distressed, rather than easing as it should, and she may then suffer an attack of wheezing which could possibly persist for half-an-hour or more.

Most asthmatic children *do* suffer from exercise asthma, and there are some asthmatics who *only* experience asthma symptoms after exercise.

It is important that you seek treatment to protect the child from further distress as soon as you or your child's teachers notice breathing difficulties occurring after exercise. If not, she will begin to associate games with feeling poorly, and will then, quite understandably, try to avoid these activities whenever possible.

Your doctor will almost certainly recognise the symptoms when told that wheezing comes on *after* exercise. He may then want to confirm his diagnosis by carrying out a simple breathing test with your child after exercise, and perhaps again following treatment, to evaluate the improvement.

Only thirty years ago, asthmatics thought that sports were out of the question as far as they were concerned, but today, thanks to the excellent treatments available, it is difficult to pinpoint a sport, even at international level, in which there is not at least one asthmatic competing. General fitness, gained by a lifestyle of sensible diet and regular exercise, is just as important for an asthmatic as for anyone else.

So, what are these liberating medications?

## 1   *Bronchodilators*

These are inhaled drugs which open up, or dilate, the bronchial tubes. They are both safe and extremely effective. The small size of the aerosol canister or rotahaler device used to administer them slips easily into a pocket, making them as convenient to use as a handkerchief.

Exercise asthma can be prevented by taking one or two puffs of a bronchodilator *before* exercise. Should the wheeze break through during the sport, another puff can be taken to relieve the wheeze and prevent further trouble.

There are bronchodilator medicines which are taken by mouth. Theophylins (such as Phyllocontin or Slo-Phyllin), taken regularly, can reduce or eliminate exercise asthma symptoms.

Most asthmatics who suffer from exercise asthma carry an inhaler to use during sports, as their doctors direct, for 'on the spot' relief.

Here is a list of bronchodilators which can be used in pressurised aerosol inhalers before exercise:

| Approved Name | Proprietary Name |
|---|---|
| Fenoterol | Berotec |
| Isoprenaline | Medihaler-Iso |
| Orciprenaline | Alupent |
| Pirbuterol | Exirel |
| Reproterol | Bronchodil |
| Rimeterol | Pulmadil |
| Salbutamol | Ventolin |
| | Cobutolin |
| | Salbulin |
| Terbutaline | Bricanyl |

## 2   *Sodium Cromoglycate (Intal)*

Intal is not a bronchodilator. It lessens the sensitivity of the airways when taken regularly over a period of time. However, it is effective in preventing exercise asthma when taken just before exercise, again by means of an aerosol spray or spinhaler device. It will *not* relieve an exercise-induced wheeze once it has started. If this happens, an inhaled bronchodilator should give speedy relief.

Some asthmatics find that regular use of Intal is the only treatment they need to prevent exercise-induced asthma.

## 3   *Corticosteroid Inhalers (Becotide and Bextasol)*

Like Intal, these inhalers are unable to provide instant relief from wheezing. Unlike Intal or a bronchodilator, these inhalers do not give any protection against exercise-induced asthma when taken just before exercise. They are preventative treatments which need to be taken regularly over a period of time before they become effective.

Once this sort of regime is established, these inhalers can be helpful in controlling exercise-induced asthma. If wheezing does break through during exercise, it is quite safe to use an inhaled bronchodilator as well.

The most important thing to remember is that, although these aerosols are very useful in enabling asthmatics to participate fully in sporting activities, bronchodilator aerosols are intended to relieve mild to moderate asthmatic conditions and, should they prove insufficient or the benefit derived from them not last, then medical assistance *must* be sought.

Some young children encounter problems when trying to use their inhalers correctly. In some instances, they may be helped by a simple, lightweight device called a nebuhaler. This will enable them to maximise the efficiency of their aerosol medication. The dose from the aerosol is released into the nebuhaler, rather than straight into the child's mouth. Because the drug particles remain suspended in the air inside the nebuhaler's chamber, while a valve prevents them from escaping, the child's inspiration does not have to coincide with the single critical moment when the pressurised dose is released from the canister. Instead, two or three breaths can be taken from the nebuhaler mouthpiece in the child's own time. Even a child so young as to be unable to co-ordinate his breathing well enough to use a pressurised aerosol efficiently, can be taught to use a nebuhaler.

A tube spacer inhaler is a similar though smaller, sometimes collapsible, device. It is slightly less efficient than the nebuhaler, but useful nonetheless, because it is scarcely larger than the canister itself and so conveniently portable.

Unfortunately, the nebuhaler is not compatible with all pressurised aerosols. It may be used with Pulmicort (a steroid inhaler) and Bricanyl (a bronchodilator), and is also suitable for use with the Intal aerosol. But Ventolin, Becotide and Bextasol do not fit into the nebuhaler, and even if they did, the nebuhaler is too small to cope efficiently with the size of the cloud of mist which these canisters produce.

Your doctor will be able to determine which treatment, or combination of treatments, will be the most beneficial to your child. Once this has been established, she should be encouraged to take part in all the sports she enjoys. The main thing to remember is that wheezing due to exercise does *not* mean that the particular activity must be abandoned permanently, but it does indicate that treatment or additional treatment may be necessary to allow your child to enjoy her sports unhindered.

There are some sports which are said to be more easily tolerated than others. These are the types of sport which require short bursts of effort rather than sustained endurance. Sprinting rather than cross-country running, cricket rather than football. It is difficult to reconcile this totally against the weight of evidence which seems to demonstrate, quite clearly thanks to our record-breaking athletes with asthma, that *any* sport is possible, if fitness is built up steadily and the most effective treatment taken properly under the direction of your doctor.

## Asthma: All in the Mind?

At one time asthma was considered to be largely a nervous disorder. Unfortunately, this misapprehension still prevails today, largely because so little information is readily available about the disease, except to those closely involved. Hence the old image of frail, sensitive folk, manipulating those around them by self-inducement of frightening attacks, lives on for many people, however diluted in the telling.

No one is yet totally sure why some people suffer from

asthma. It is rather like a large jigsaw, almost complete, yet with a few pieces still missing.

It has been proved that asthma occurs more frequently in those children whose parents or other close relatives have suffered from asthma. On the other hand, the large majority of children born to asthmatic parents have no chest problems at all.

Children with asthma are vulnerable to certain conditions which leave their peers completely unaffected. The asthmatic child, when exposed to allergens, exercise, infection or stress, displays any or all of the typical symptoms of asthma: wheezing, coughing, breathlessness. This is because the small muscles which surround the airways of the lungs tighten, making the airways narrower, and so restrict the flow of air. You may hear this being referred to as bronchoconstriction. This tightening of the small muscles is accompanied by swelling of the inner lining of the tubes and by an outpouring of secretions, which makes breathing even more difficult.

So, asthma is a very real physical condition, but as in many other illnesses—perhaps the prime example is a severe heart condition—stress or anxiety can certainly make matters worse. Think what happens when you have a fright: your heart beats faster, you become breathless and you might even faint. If you are worried about something your body becomes tense, and it is only a matter of time before those tight muscles begin to hurt. If, on the other hand, you are happy and relaxed, aches and pains miraculously fade away as you turn your mind to other things.

An asthmatic responds to stress exactly the same as anyone else, but his lungs are his weakest line of defence and so show the effects of the tension first—and in a way that is hard to miss. It is noisy and he is obviously distressed, but that does not make him any more or less neurotic than somebody with a stiff neck.

Human beings, being the contradictory folk they are, can also confound the scientist when unexpected results turn up during controlled tests. Asthmatics who are allergic, for example, to cats or grass, have been known to start wheezing at the very sight of a picture of a cat or a field. Scientifically impossible, perhaps, yet it happens.

The quite understandable anxiety an asthmatic might feel, upon discovering that he has left his asthma medicine at home, might precipitate an attack, and an asthmatic child might try to work himself up into an attack in order to get his own way, miss school or whatever. First of all, get to the bottom of it. Do not be too busy or leave it until later. Is it just plain naughtiness? The odd temper tantrum, however unreasonable, is, as all parents are only too well aware, perfectly normal. We all have our own way of dealing with them. My own daughter is left to get on with it by herself—having first been transported to her own room if necessary. She usually calms down pretty quickly; it is so boring being a prima donna on one's own. I do not need to tell you how best to deal with your own child's temper. Is there something more behind it? Bullying at school? Unable to keep up with her work? Personality clash with the teacher? Loathing of games? Unhappy about something in the home?

Talk, care, root it out. Those sorts of problems can be overcome. If there is not a specific problem and the asthma-inducing tantrums are ruining your life, you need help. Do not wait until you become ill, too, or until you lose your temper and strike the child; go for help. Doctors have come across most things before, and it is certainly no sign of weakness on your part to try to share the load; it is simply common sense. A family must be a team and one member of that team cannot be allowed to disrupt the lives of everyone else. Besides which, if things are extremely bad, it is up to you to help, because a child just does not know how to help herself.

## Steroids

A steroid medication is a powerful hormone drug used to treat asthma when symptoms are not being controlled sufficiently by the patient's usual treatment. Steroids are actually manufactured naturally in our bodies. The Corticosteroids, Cortisone and Hydrocortisone, are produced by the outer part or 'cortex' of the adrenal glands. All other steroids used in asthma are synthetic.

Steroids appear under a bewildering array of trade names:

| Proper Name | Trade Names |
|---|---|
| BECLOMETHASONE | Becotide (Aerosol), Aldecin (Aus) |
| BETAMETHASONE | Betnelan, Betnesol, Bextasol (Aerosol), Celestone (Aus USA) |
| CORTISONE | Cortelan, Cortisab, Cortisyl, Cortate (Aus), Cortone (USA) |
| DEXAMETHASONE | Decasdron, Dexacortisyl, Oradexon, Dexone (USA), Dexmethsone (Aus) |
| HYDROCORTISONE | Efcortelan, Efcortisol, Hydrocortisab, Hydrocortone, Solu-Cortef, Eldecort (USA), Cetacort (Aus) |
| METHYL-PREDNISOLONE | Depo-Medrone, Medro-Cortex, Medrone, Solu-Medrone, Medrol (Aus USA) |
| PARAMETHASONE | Haldrate, Metilar |
| PREDNISONE and PREDNISOLONE | Codelcortone, Codelsol, Decortisyl, Delta-Cortef, Delta-Cortril, Deltacortone, Deltastab, Di-Adreson, Precortisyl, Prednesol, Sintisone, Ultra cortenol, Deltasolone (Aus), Prelone (Aus), Meticortelone (USA) |

TRIAMCINOLONE             Adcortyl, Kenalog, Ledercort,
                          Lederspan, Triamacin (USA),
                          Kenalone (Aus)

When steroids are given in large doses over a period of time, they reduce the body's natural production of steroids. These are essential to life, so one can see how dangerous it would be suddenly to withdraw the medically approved dose. Your doctor will have determined the length of the course most appropriate to control an attack, and you will notice that the dose is reduced gradually, allowing the body time to readjust and begin its own steroid production once again.

Most courses are short, i.e. three to seven days, and the child's usual treatment, e.g. Intal, Ventolin, etc., should be maintained at the same time. This will not only help to prevent the asthma from breaking through again once the course is finished, but will also help to keep the dose of steroids down to a minimum.

Sometimes the asthma symptoms return once the course of steroids has been completed; another course may then be necessary. This is not a cause for alarm, unless the courses must be repeated time after time and have become continuous. If this happens, and all other treatment proves inadequate, your doctor may suggest that your child takes a low-dose steroid therapy by mouth every other day. Side effects are rare when this sort of regime is established, even over long periods of time—years rather than weeks. The body appears to correct itself on the days between treatment, so do not shy away from this form of medication if it proves to be the only way to control your child's asthma.

Tablets should be swallowed during or after meals, but can be taken at any time during an emergency. Some tablets have a special coating to prevent stomach upsets, and there are also soluble steroid tablets available.

It is important to ensure that any child who is taking large doses of steroids by mouth carries a Steroid Card or wears a Medic-Alert bracelet. You can obtain a Medic-Alert bracelet from the following address: Medic-Alert Foundation, 11 Clifton Terrace, London N4. (Tel: 01-263 8596). If for any reason she has to be admitted to hospital for treatment, it is essential that the medical team are aware that your child is taking steroids. This is because, should surgery be necessary, or if a severe infection is present, the body needs more Cortisone than usual. If the adrenal glands are not functioning at full capacity because Cortisone is being taken by mouth, the doctors will need to give their patient extra Cortisone to compensate for this shortfall.

You may hear doctors referring to topical steroids and systemic steroids. Systemic steroids are those taken either by mouth or injection. They dissolve in the body water and so are carried round the whole body. Hydrocortisone can be injected into either a muscle or a vein as a single injection, or is sometimes given in hospital through a drip. There is a 'slow release' form of injected steroid available which can give relief for several weeks. It is not used to control persistent asthma symptoms, but can be used for the hay fever type of asthma symptoms. This has not proved to be more useful than taking a small daily dose of steroid tablets during the most difficult months.

Topical steroids *do not* dissolve in the body water, so only have an effect upon a particular part of the body, e.g. the lungs, when treatment is given with an inhaled steroid medication such as Becotide or Bextasol. Even though regular small doses of inhaled steroids can produce quite large concentrations of the drug exactly at the point where it is needed, barely any is absorbed by the rest of the body. Thus, this is the safest way to use steroids in asthma.

In order to derive maximum benefit from this form of treatment, it is important that the inhaler is used correctly.

Particularly with the pressurised aerosol canister, it is worth making sure that it is not being used in the casual way in which you might use a pressurised can of mouth freshener.

1   Shake the canister and remove the cap.
2   Breathe out gently.
3   Close the mouth tightly around the mouthpiece. Just as the breath begins to be slowly drawn in again, press the canister.
4   When the breath is fully drawn, it should be held for about 5 to 10 seconds.
5   Breathe out again . . . slowly.

If the prescribed dose is two blasts, wait about one minute before taking the second. An inhaled bronchodilator should be expected to bring relief after approximately two minutes.

Some people prefer to use a rotahaler. This is a small plastic device which, when twisted sharply, breaks open a small capsule of dry powder which may then be inhaled through the mouthpiece. A much sharper intake of breath is required to draw the powder out of this device, but the breath must still be held for the same five to ten seconds. It will probably be necessary to take two or three breaths before the powder disappears completely, but at least you can easily open the device to check whether it has all been inhaled.

If asthma symptoms are troublesome at the time when these inhaled steroids are due to be taken, try using a bronchodilator first to 'open up' the airways. Remember, too, that steroids take some time to become effective; you cannot use them to obtain instant relief from asthma symptoms. Use a bronchodilator for this purpose.

Doctors sometimes refer to regular steroid therapy, e.g. with Becotide or Bextasol inhalers, as prophylactic treatment. This simply means preventative treatment.

Steroids do not cure asthma, but they are able to control distressing symptoms and can be life-saving at critical times. No one knows exactly how they help to control asthmatic wheezing, but the major function of steroid medicines is to decrease swelling, inflammation or redness wherever they may appear in the body, and for whatever reason. Mucosal inflammation will not respond to bronchodilators. Corticosteroids are needed to reduce this, so removing the obstruction.

*Side Effects*
These are virtually non existent with inhaled steroids. They can only touch the mouth, throat or windpipe on their journey to the lungs. The only possible side effect would be a minor throat irritation, or an infection in the mouth called thrush. These are extremely unlikely to occur and can be treated quite easily with throat lozenges. One simple precaution to be taken after each dose of an inhaled steroid, to help prevent thrush, is to wash the mouth out thoroughly.

I have noticed that when Sara leaves hospital following an acute attack, having been given a week's supply of Prednisolone (steroid) tablets to take at home, she is extremely excitable for the duration of the course. Thankfully, all returns to normal shortly after she stops taking the tablets.

When steroid tablets are needed month after month on a *daily* basis, they can cause side effects. Any one of the following *may* occur:

1   Weight gain, due to:
 a   Increased appetite, which can be controlled to some extent by educating the child so that she recognises and enjoys the less fattening foods—also ensuring that her diet is as varied and interesting as possible.

b   Water retention. If this is severe enough to cause swelling of the ankles or high blood pressure, diuretics or 'water tablets' can be prescribed by your doctor to remove the excess.

2   Increased hairiness of the body or face.

3   Conversely, in our experience with our daughter, hair loss.

4   Rounding of the face, commonly known as 'moon face'.

5   Hump-like swelling on the back of the neck.

6   Skin bruises easily.

7   Acne.

8   Abdominal pains. Bloating.

9   Temporary rise in blood sugar.

10   Mild to marked decrease in growth rate. Providing the child is young enough to continue growing, a sudden spurt would almost certainly occur if the treatment was decreased or stopped altogether, allowing her to make up the lost growth.

11   Excess perspiration. Flushed face.

12   Dry mouth.

13   Fatigue.

14   Leg cramps.

15   Sleeping difficulties.

16   Although extremely rare and usually found in adult patients who have been on continuous systemic steroid therapy for more than one year, bones may become thin resulting in painful fractures.

17   Cortisone may mask other infections, making the patient feel quite well when in fact she may be suffering from a serious infection such as pneumonia. Therefore, it is essential that anyone taking steroids by mouth should receive regular check-ups from her doctor.

When administered properly under supervision, steroids rarely cause these side effects. Do not be afraid to use them under the careful direction of your doctor, when other forms of treatment have proved ineffectual. Remember that inhaled steroid preparations, with their minimal risk of side effects, are of immense value, allowing many asthmatics who have had to take steroid tablets over long periods of time, either to greatly reduce the dose of these or even to find them altogether unnecessary.

## Will My Child grow out of Asthma?

There is not a doctor alive today who will give you a written guarantee on this question. It is possible to quote probabilities and statistics but, sadly, these are notoriously unreliable. It is said that a child who has been breast-fed is more likely to be asthma-free in adult life than one who has not.

There is a particularly unpleasant viral infection called acute bronchiolitis. This illness occurs in the first months of life and may render the airways abnormally sensitive for several years. This may account for the fact that wheezing occurs so frequently in young children who do not appear to have any allergies. This sort of wheezing would be unlikely to continue into adult life.

Wheezing in children under five years old usually occurs when they have an infection such as the common cold. By the age of seven, they have built up some immunity to this sort of everyday virus infection and so are less likely to wheeze. Again, the future for these children looks bright. They, too, would be less likely to grow into asthmatic adults.

Things do not look quite so rosy for the allergic child with asthma. It is still possible that she may grow out of her asthma, but perhaps rather later, in her teens. The best you can do is help her to avoid the things which 'trigger' her asthma. The less trouble she has with asthma as a child, the more likely she is to grow out of it.

Some children have an allergy to common dust, known as atopy. Atopic children with asthma may also have other allergies, and a few may have developed eczema as babies, suffering that dreadfully itchy skin condition which often shows itself most obviously in the folds of the elbows, the wrists and behind the knees. Unfortunately, these children stand less chance of growing out of their asthma.

Chances are reduced, too, for the child who suffers persistent, chronic attacks which require many hospital admissions.

Very occasionally, those children who appear to have overcome their asthma as they grow older, suffer an unexpected and most unwelcome return of their symptoms in adult life. This might be because of an infection, or due to stress. These recurrences only happen to about one third of those who have wheezed as children.

Although the fact remains that no one can be certain who will or will not grow out of asthma, there is no reason why your child should not be one of the lucky ones.

## Questions and Answers

*Are some places better than others for an asthmatic to live?*
First of all, do not be misled if you are told, 'This is a very bad place for asthmatics.' Sadly, asthma is such a common disease that this statement could apply to almost any-where.

Obviously, an asthmatic who suffered from a pollen-induced condition would be advised to avoid close proximity to the open countryside or other densely vegetated areas. Yet, because asthma is such a very individual problem, it would be both impossible and wrong to generalise.

An asthmatic living in a highly industrialised setting might complain, with some justification, that the smoky atmosphere was bad for her chest. But say, for instance, members of an asthmatic's family smoke indoors, then the wrong sort of environment would be created wherever she lived.

Low-lying, damp places would not be beneficial, but

think, too, about the strenuous exercise involved if you choose a hilly location, not to mention the possible increased exposure to windy conditions.

Narrowing it down to a choice of home, much against my own personal preference, we would always choose a modern type of house, guaranteed to be free from damp and unnecessary dust, rather than a more appealing, but possibly asthma-provoking, older property.

*Can hypnotism play a part in the treatment of asthma?*
Although used infrequently, hypnotism can occasionally aid an asthmatic by enabling her, through self-hypnosis, to induce a relaxed state whenever an attack threatens. Apart from the obvious drawback that it is not always possible to anticipate the attack in sufficient time for the hypnosis to become effective, where you happen to be at the time must also be relevant. I can see that hypnotism, used to induce a state of relaxation while at the same time remaining *totally* aware, would have its uses, but, personally, I would rather keep my wits about me in order to make certain I was monitoring the condition accurately.

*If we went to Switzerland on holiday, to what height could our asthmatic child safely go?*
High altitudes are known to suit asthmatics, possibly because so few house dust mites are able to survive in the dry, clean atmosphere. There is certainly little or no pollution. Many high Swiss resorts such as Arosa and Davos have the reputation of being beneficial to severely affected asthmatics. If you choose to go skiing in the winter season, take the precaution of giving your child her prescribed medication before she goes out into the cold, just as you would see that she takes the same medication before exercise. The simple precaution of keeping a scarf over her mouth for a while will enable her to breathe in warmer, moist air, at least until she becomes accustomed to

the dramatic change in temperature when leaving the heated lodge or hotel and going out into the crisp mountain air.

*If you suffered from asthma as a child and then go for a very long time without having any symptoms, would it still be possible to have a recurrence?*
It is always possible that there might be a recurrence, but this is by no means a certainty. Anyone, at any age, can suffer from asthma, whether or not he or she was asthmatic as a child.

*Is it true that asthma, hay fever, eczema and migraine are related?*
Genetically, migraine is not related to asthma, hay fever and eczema. Like asthma, migraine can be triggered by food and drink—such as red wine.

*If a parent has migraine, could a child inherit one of the other complaints, such as asthma, hay fever or eczema?*
Because migraine is not genetically related to the others it would not be possible for a child to inherit one of the other conditions because her parent has migraine. However, like the others, migraine can be passed on through the family.

*Is goat's milk helpful in an asthmatic's diet?*
If cow's milk provokes symptoms, whether they be asthmatic or eczematous, goat's milk is hardly ever shown to be a better alternative. It is more expensive than cow's milk and may not be pasteurised.

*Is asthma curable?*
Asthma is controllable. A cure is still being sought.

*Is allergy part of the syllabus for medical students in medical schools, and if so, to what extent?*
Although only a few medical schools have allergy clinics

which cover the subject broadly, allergy must impinge on all the subjects which a student covers during training.

*If a mother breast-feeds her baby, knowing that this will help to reduce the risk of allergies such as asthma, must she stop drinking cow's milk?*
No.

*What are the side effects of Ventolin?*
In about 10 per cent of patients, Ventolin has been found to cause a slight muscular tremor when taken in tablet or syrup form. This percentage would also apply to Ventolin given by injection or in a drip. Ventolin atomisers direct their beneficial effect to where it is needed, the lungs, and they are very safe.

*What is the earliest age at which a diagnosis of asthma can be made?*
After the age of one year, although doctors still differ in their diagnosis of asthma.

*What allergies cause attacks?*
There is no known substance which has not been found to have the potential to cause an asthma attack in somebody.

*Should sports centres have oxygen available to aid distressed asthmatics?*
Although oxygen is used as part of the treatment during a severe attack, this is generally in hospital or under the supervision of a GP. An asthmatic would usually be carrying her own medication in the form of a small inhaler if she anticipated problems during exercise. This should be the first action to take. If she fails to respond quickly to this medication, she should be taken to the nearest hospital's Casualty Department without delay.

*Are skin tests worthwhile for a 'wheezy' child and do they help?*
Although not absolutely reliable, skin tests do help to identify those children who are suffering from some types

of allergic asthma, e.g. summer bronchitis may in fact be pollen-induced asthma. However, they will not identify those allergies that are caused by food and drink, or symptoms caused by inhaling such things as cigarette smoke. The skin tests themselves do nothing to improve an asthmatic condition, other than by their limited ability to identify some of the possible triggers responsible for that condition.

*Should we have more children if we already have one asthmatic?*
Because asthma does tend to run in families, there is going to be a greater risk for those parents who already have one asthmatic child. That risk is a small one. Asthma *is* controllable and the fact that you already have an asthmatic child will enable you to identify any potential problems at the earliest time, which may be brought under control before they cause distress.

*I am 24 and have had asthma since childhood. Recently, I started running and find that my general health and state of mind has improved greatly. Although I take Intal regularly, I find that I cannot run for any length of time unless I also take Ventolin beforehand. Am I doing myself any harm?*
This is exactly the way in which asthmatic athletes, Olympic medallists among them, manage their asthma. It is certainly not harmful.

*Do breathing exercises help?*
Breathing exercises which are used to promote calm and relaxation do help to a certain extent, but, some exercises which were recommended in the past have been shown, by scientific tests, to be not only ineffective but also potentially harmful. This is due to the fact that they were based on a wrong idea. During an asthma attack the bronchial tubes contract, so the asthmatic breathes with his chest expanded as much as possible so as to hold the tubes as wide open as

he can. As he breathes out, the tubes tend to close. Doctors thought that this expanded position of the chest was bad for asthmatics and so exercises were designed to teach them to breathe out as much as possible. It is now known that this would only make breathing more difficult. These exercises should not be used. Some asthmatics adopt a stooped position; this is undesirable. Certainly, in this case, proper breathing exercises would help to improve their posture.

*When my daughter has short courses of steroids (regular daily medicine Intal and Ventolin), is this the same type of steroid that is supposed to cause metabolic imbalance in athletes?*
The steroids that athletes take are Anabolic steroids and *not* the steroids given to asthmatics.

*Shall I have to take drugs for ever?*
This depends both on age and what sort of drugs are being taken. Many children who lose their asthma as teenagers, or even earlier, will be able to stop taking their medications. However, there is always the possibility that their asthma might recur later in life, necessitating a return to some form of medication. For those who develop asthma as adults, the outlook is not so optimistic. They may well have to continue treatment for the rest of their lives, unless there is an occupational or environmental cause for their asthma which can be removed or avoided.

*My GP is simply not interested. What should I do?*
Ask him to refer you to a chest consultant. If he refuses, go to your local hospital's Casualty Department and see the casualty officer. He will be able to help by referring you to a consultant, and between them they should be able to recommend at least one GP who *is* interested in asthma. You must then ask this GP if it is possible to join his practice. If he agrees, you must ask the Local Executive

Council (telephone number and address in the telephone directory, or ask at your local library or Citizens' Advice Bureau) to transfer your NHS records from your old to your new doctor.

*What should I do if my inhaler does not work?*
If it is a new one take it back to the chemist and explain your problem. If it is empty, you have allowed yourself to become careless if you have not got a replacement. The management of asthma brings with it many responsibilities which you cannot afford to overlook. Your regular chemist might be understanding and solve the problem for you, but it would be better to ensure that you always have at least one back-up inhaler in reserve.

*We are about to buy a new house. Do some forms of central heating cause more problems than others?*
Under-floor heating does exacerbate dust allergy, but other types of heating do not.

*We are thinking of buying a house which has cavity-wall insulation, but have heard that this may be harmful to asthma sufferers. What should we do?*
These problems are caused when the insulation is new. When first installed, fumes from some types of insulation, such as those containing formaldehyde or formalin, may cause adverse reactions and not only for asthma sufferers. Symptoms may include running eyes, nose, even nausea. These fumes should evaporate in due course and would then only continue to cause problems if the outer skin containing the insulation was cracked.

*My hay fever symptoms bear no relation at all to the broadcast pollen count; I can feel terrible when the count is low and fine when the count is high. Why is this?*
Most pollen counts are issued to the media in the morning

and will not appear in the press until the following morning, so they could not possibly reflect your condition. Radio and television are more immediate, but even they are referring to the pollen in the air during the past 24 hours, and regional variations may differ enormously.

*Is it safe to have my asthmatic child immunised?*
Any chest infection may bring on an asthma attack, or make an existing spasm worse. This makes it doubly important to protect your asthmatic child from two unpleasant infections which can both harm the lungs: whooping cough and measles.

Although vaccines to prevent these illnesses have been available for many years, some doctors are still unwilling to give them to asthmatic children, especially those who also suffer from eczema. This view is mistaken; it is most important that these children are immunised.

Whooping cough can be particularly dangerous for asthmatic children. It is an infection of the airways in the lungs. The symptoms are extremely unpleasant, as any parent who has witnessed them will know. The prolonged, racking coughing fits may well cause the child to vomit and can often make a young child turn blue, or even, in the worst circumstances, stop breathing. Whooping cough has also been known to cause brain damage and fatalities have occurred, although these are rare. Vaccination to prevent whooping cough is usually started between three and four months of age and has to be repeated twice at four to six-week intervals. Because this injection also guards against tetanus and diphtheria, it is commonly known as the 'triple vaccine'. A few children do react to the whooping cough part of the injection. This reaction will show itself as a mild fever and possibly soreness at the site of the injection; it may be expected to last for two to three days.

Proof has not yet been found to show that the whooping cough vaccine can cause permanent brain damage. If a small risk should exist, and doctors estimate that one in 300,000 might possibly be so affected, the risk from brain damage incurred by leaving a child unvaccinated, and so liable to catch whooping cough, is far greater.

The Department of Health has recommended that some children should not be immunised against whooping cough. These are:

1   Those with a parent, brother or sister who has epilepsy. Fits affecting more distant relatives do not count.
2   Children who have already had a convulsion.
3   Children who have had signs of brain damage previously, usually in the first few days of life.
4   Children who have had a severe reaction to a previous injection.
5   Children who have a temperature at the time of one of the injections.

Children with asthma, eczema or other forms of allergy can be vaccinated as safely as any other children, apart from those classified above. The injections can be given even when the child has an obvious asthma attack with coughing and wheezing. In the past, children with asthma symptoms have not been immunised. This was quite wrong, for wheezing does not make a reaction more likely.

Measles is a highly infectious virus and, although it does not last as long as whooping cough, it is also extremely unpleasant. Nearly always affecting the lungs, measles can also cause brain damage in about one in 1000 cases. The vaccine available today is extremely effective and requires only one injection, when the child is between 12 and 15 months old. This vaccine has no effect whatsoever on the brain. Again, there has been some reluctance to give this vaccine to allergic children, most particularly to those who suffer from an allergy to eggs or egg products. This is simply because the vaccine used to be grown in hens' eggs and consequently contained a small quantity of egg.

Nowadays, the vaccines are grown on cultures of cells from the chicks and so do not contain these egg traces.

It is better not to give the measles vaccine to those children who suffer extreme reactions when they eat egg or egg products—reactions such as swelling of the face or skin or acute breathlessness; some, indeed, may even collapse if they ingest the smallest trace of egg. The vaccine should not be given to children if they are sick with a fever; neither should it be given to a child who is receiving steroid medications, either by mouth in tablet form, or by injection, for these will reduce the child's ability to respond properly to the vaccine. Children taking inhaled steroids (Becotide, Bextasol, Pulmicort) can be immunised quite safely.

Children who suffer a worsening of their asthma or eczema, or those who suffer from diarrhoea or vomiting when they eat egg, may also be immunised.

Asthmatic children should be allowed to benefit from all the routine immunisations which are available to them. These include tetanus, diphtheria, poliomyelitis, and later, in adolescence, the BCG for tuberculosis and, for girls, german measles. However, it should be noted that both the BCG and german measles vaccines are live and should not be given to any child who is receiving steroids by mouth or injection. For those who suffer from acute symptoms requiring steroid treatment, an influenza vaccine is also a good precaution.

Some other injections may be needed if travel to tropical countries is planned. These are also safe for an asthmatic child; for instance, TAB (typhoid and paratyphoid), cholera and yellow fever. Again, yellow fever is a live vaccine and must not be given to a child on any type of systemic steroid therapy.

# Organisations

**The Asthma Society and Friends of the Asthma
Research Council**
At the time of writing, the Asthma Society is supporting 28
separate research projects throughout Great Britain.

When you become a member of the Friends of the
Asthma Research Council, you will receive the Society's
annual report, which includes information about the
various projects. These cannot fail to be of interest to those
closely involved with the disease. I have always found it a
great stimulus to my optimism, to know that the funds are
being put to such a positive and determined use.

There are almost 130 local branches of the Friends of the
Asthma Research Council throughout the country, all of
whom are striving for wider recognition and understanding
of asthma. Far from being dry, introspective societies, they
make vigorous efforts to go out and inform the general
public about asthma, and you only have to read one of the
Asthma Research Council's news sheets to understand
that these are the energetic tentacles of a great organisation.
Most of the branches offer a varied social calendar and
pursue fund-raising campaigns with unflagging enthusiasm.
Activities include swimming clubs, sponsored swims,
marathons, talks, wine tastings and fashion shows—the
list could go on and on. Two of the facets which I personally
want to stress are, first and perhaps most important, if you

need support, understanding and help, you will find it at your local branch, and, secondly, they all appear to have a great deal of fun. The Asthma Society arranges outward bound courses at Eskdale in the Lake District, the Kielder Adventure Centre in Northumberland and at Cotton College on the edge of the Peak District. Young people whose asthma is well controlled, but who perhaps would not undertake such adventurous activities, are enabled to do so, as each course is under the supervision of a doctor.

Taking a retrospective view of Sara's asthma in all its harrowing detail, it is quite natural that I should feel more confident now that her dreadful symptoms are being successfully controlled, but this is a form of complacency which I must eschew. What parent wants her child to remain indefinitely on such a programme of drugs? What we need and must have is a *cure* for asthma. This will only be found through painstaking, time-consuming, *expensive* research. The Asthma Research Council needs constant funding to keep the ball rolling.

It is harder to feel the same level of commitment to support such an organisation once your own crisis has passed, but if *your* child is one of the lucky ones who sloughs off her asthma as she grows to maturity, never forget how she used to be and always remember the children who are still suffering.

Only your sustained compassion and generosity will provide the Asthma Research Council with the life-blood it needs to continue its most important work. As well as support from your local branch, you can obtain practical advice, set out clearly in pamphlet form on a number of topics associated with asthma from: The Asthma Society and Friends of the Asthma Research Council, 300 Upper Street, London N1 2XX. (Tel: 01-226 2260)

They will also direct you to your local branch, and are pleased to see visitors at the London office. Needless to say, new members are always most welcome—who knows, you may even feel ready one day to open your own local branch!

## Organisations Overseas

*Australia*

Asthma Association Citizens' Advice Bureau (ACT), Tel: Canberra 886088.

Asthma Foundation of New South Wales (AWS), 1 Angel Place, Sydney, New South Wales 2000.

Asthma Foundation of Queensland, PO Box 122, East Brisbane, Queensland 4169.

Asthma Foundation of Southern Australia, 33 Pirie Street, Adelaide, Southern Australia 5000.

Asthma Foundation of Tasmania, 82 Hapden Road, Battery Point, Hobart, Tasmania 7000.

Asthma Foundation of Victoria, 2 Highfield Grove, Kew, Victoria 3101.

Asthma Foundation of Western Australia Inc, 61 Heytesbury Road, Subiaco, Western Australia 6008.

*Ireland*

Asthma Society of Ireland, 24 Anglesea Street, Dublin 2. (Tel: 01-716551)

*Canada*

Asthma Society of Canada, Box 213, Stn. K, Toronto, Ontario, M4P 2G5.

*New Zealand*

Asthma Foundation of New Zealand, Secretary, PO Box 1459, Wellington.

*United States of America*

Asthma Care Association of America, PO Box 568, Spring Valley Road, Ossining, NY 10562. (Tel: (914) 762-1941)

Asthmatic Children's Foundation of New York, PO Box 568, Spring Valley Road, Ossining, NY 10562. (Tel: (212) 355-2872)

National Foundation for Asthma, PO Box 30069, Tucson, AZ 85751. (Tel: (602) 323-6046)

# Glossary

Words you may hear used in connection with asthma.

ADRENALINE     A drug used as a bronchodilator (see BRONCHODILATOR). Given by injection in the treatment of acute attacks of asthma. It is produced naturally in the body during emotional stress.

ALLERGEN     A substance inducing an allergic state or reaction, e.g. pollen, house dust, animal dander (skin dust), mould spores, certain foods.

ALLERGIC     Having an allergy.

ALLERGY     Abnormal sensitivity to a specific substance.

AMINOPHYLLINE     An anti-asthma drug given as tablets, suppositories or injection.

ANAPHYLAXIS     A rapid and serious type of allergic reaction caused by further exposure to the same original allergen.

ALVEOLI     Microscopic air sacs in the lungs.

ANTIBIOTIC     A substance which destroys or stops the growth of harmful bacteria.

| | |
|---|---|
| ANTIBODIES | Substances in the body occurring naturally or by exposure to an antigen, which tend to combine with the antigen or allergen (see ANTIGEN and ALLERGEN). |
| ANTIGEN | An enzyme or toxin to which the body reacts by producing antibodies. |
| ANTIHISTAMINE | Prevents histamine reacting with the smooth muscle. Unfortunately, although antihistamines are very effective in controlling hay fever symptoms, they have disappointing results as far as childhood asthma is concerned. |
| ASTHMA | A chronic disorder characterised by wheezing, coughing, difficulty in breathing and a suffocating feeling. |
| ASTHMATIC | A person who suffers from asthma. |
| ASTHMATIC BRONCHITIS | A form of asthma (see WHEEZY BRONCHITIS). |
| BACTERIA | Typically one-celled micro-organisms which have no chlorophyll. These multiply by simple division and occur in various forms. Some cause disease, but others are necessary for life. |
| BASOPHILS | White blood cells, very similar to tissue mast cells. |
| BECOTIDE | A topical (inhaled) steroid medication. |
| BEXTASOL | Another topical (inhaled) steroid medication. |
| BLOCKING ANTIBODY | A type of antibody produced arti- |

ficially in the body during a course
of desensitisation (see DESENSITIS-
ATION), so called because it is be-
lieved to act by blocking the
activity of allergens (see ALLER-
GEN).

BRONCHI
The two main branches of the
trachea or windpipe.

BRONCHO
Meaning to have to do with the
bronchi.

BRONCHOCONSTRICTION
When the small muscles around
the airways tighten, making the
airways narrower and so restrict-
ing the flow of air.

BRONCHODILATOR
A substance which makes wider,
dilates, the bronchial tubes.

BRONCHIOLES
Small airways leading off from
the bronchi.

BRONCHITIS
An inflammation of the mucous
lining of the bronchial tubes.

BRONCHUS
Either one of the two main
branches of the trachea or windpipe.

CANDIDIASIS
See THRUSH.

CHILDISH WHEEZING
A form of asthma.

CODEINE
Found in many cough prep-
arations. Useful to relieve dry,
recurrent night-time cough associated with infection. This is
not desirable for asthma patients
because it can interfere with normal breathing and sometimes aggravate asthma.

COMPLEMENT SYSTEMS
Consists of at least 20 distinct
serum proteins concerned in different kinds of inflammation, in-

cluding release of histamine in an allergic reaction.

CONTRA INDICATION — Negative aspect. (Literal meaning: against sign.)

CONSTRICT — To contract; make smaller or narrower.

CONSTRICTION — Feeling of tightness or pressure; as in the chest.

CONSULTANT — A doctor who specialises in a particular branch of medicine.

CORTISONE — An adrenal gland hormone (steroid) used in treating asthma.

CYANOSIS — A bluish coloration of the skin caused by lack of oxygen in the blood.

DESENSITISATION — The reduction of sensitivity in an allergic person. Desensitising injections are available, although as asthma is rarely due to a single cause or allergy, there are few doctors who will recommend this type of treatment.

DIAPHRAGM — The partition of muscles and tendons between the chest cavity and the abdominal cavity. Midriff.

DILATE — To make wider or larger.

DIURETICS — Water tablets. These increase the secretion and flow of urine.

DOUBLE PNEUMONIA — Pneumonia of both lungs (see PNEUMONIA).

ENTERIC — Literal meaning: intestinal. Used to describe tablets which have a protective coating to guard against stomach upsets.

EXHALATION — The act of breathing out.

FUNGI — A low-order group of plants, e.g.

mould, mildew, rusts, smuts, found in non-Polar countries. Some cause allergic reactions. They are very light and are carried away from their source for long distances in the air. It is the small fungi which cause allergy; the bigger particles being trapped by the defences in our noses and bronchial tubes. We cough and sneeze to get rid of them. The smaller ones penetrate these protective barriers and cause runny, itchy noses and eyes, or even wheezing.

GLOBULINS A group of proteins in the blood which contain most antibodies.

HAY FEVER (SEASONAL) An allergy characterised by excessive sneezing, watering and itching of the nose and eyes and blocking of the nasal passages. Caused chiefly by pollen from trees (March–May) and grasses (June and July).

HISTAMINE One of the chemicals released from the mast cells in response to allergies, exercise, emotion, infection, so causing wheezing in an asthmatic child.

HORMONE A substance formed in some organ of the body, e.g. adrenal gland, carried to another organ or tissue, where it has a specific effect. Often prepared synthetically.

HOUSEMAN A recently qualified doctor who holds a resident post in a hospital.

HOUSE DUST

A mixture of coarse and fine particles, e.g. pollen brought into the house, skin scales, hair or dried saliva of the family pet, fragments of material, bits of paper, shreds of tobacco, ash, face powder, talcum powder, dead insects, bacteria from the skin, fibres from plants, animal matter, food, debris from upholstery, curtains, carpets, rugs and stuffed toys, particles of wood from furniture, soot, mould, feathers, mites, etc.

HOUSE DUST MITE

One of the most notable causes of house dust allergy. A tiny creature just visible to the naked eye which thrives in warm, damp places.

HUMIDIFIERS

Machines which increase the level of humidity in the air. Some asthmatic children benefit from increased humidity, particularly in those homes where central heating systems create low humidity levels. However, be prepared for an increase in the humidity-loving house dust mite (another swings and roundabouts situation). I suggest you borrow and try rather than buy.

HYDROCORTISONE

An adrenal gland hormone used in treating asthma.

HYPERVENTILATE

Over-oxygenation of the blood causing dizziness and fainting, due to very rapid breathing during a severe asthma attack. (Can also be due to very deep breathing in other circumstances.)

IgE
The allergic antibody in the blood and tissues such as skin, gut, nose and lungs. Combines with an allergen, e.g. pollen, to cause an allergic reaction.

IMMUNITY
A condition where antibodies have been produced in an individual either naturally, as a response to an infection, or artificially, as a result of protective injections.

IMMUNOGLOBINS
Antibodies, e.g. IgE., IgC., IgA., IgM., formed following an antigenic stimulus.

INSPIRATION
The act of breathing in.

INTAL
Sodium Cromoglycate. A drug which acts by preventing allergic symptoms. An inhaled drug, thought to stabilise the mast cells, that is, render them less likely to release their asthma-inducing contents on stimulation. Intal is a very well-established drug, entirely safe and apparently totally without side effects. Also given for symptoms in the nose and eyes and taken by mouth for allergic symptoms in the gut.

IONISER
A machine available commercially which generates minute particles of 'ions' which cause a negative electrical charge. There is no concrete evidence that these influence the severity of a child's asthma in any way.

| | |
|---|---|
| LEUKOTRIENES | Rather similiar to histamine but 1000 times more active. Found in sputum. No drug yet available against them. |
| LUNG FUNCTION TESTS | See PEAK FLOW METER and SPIRO-METER. |
| LYMPHOCYTE | The essential cell of the immune system. |
| B-LYMPHOCYTES | When stimulated by antigen will multiply and be transformed into plasma cells. Are essential for development of humoral immune reactions. (Humoral: related to the humours of the body.) |
| T–LYMPHOCYTES | Are responsible for cellular immune reactions. The cells secrete lymphokines which affect many other cells and may act as 'killer cells'. |
| MAST CELLS | Present in the nose, lungs and skin, they include several asthma-inducing substances including histamines, which are released when stimulated either by allergic factors, exercise or emotion (see INTAL). |
| MEDIATOR | A substance which brings about a result. |
| MEDICATION | A medicine: substance used for curing, healing or relieving pain. |
| MEMBRANE | A thin, soft, pliable layer of tissue that covers or lines an organ. |
| MOON FACE | Round-faced. A possible side effect of regular long-term therapy with a systemic steroid medication. |
| MOULD | A member of the low-order plant |

group, properly known as fungi. Mould flourishes in warm, damp places. *Do not overlook vaporisers or humidifiers.* Also found in wallpaper, kapok stuffing, food storage areas, foam rubber, etc., as well as in the more expected places such as lawns, forests, compost heaps, rubbish containers, etc.

NEBUHALER  Designed for use at home in conjunction with a pressurised aerosol. The fine spray from the aerosol is released into the nebuhaler chamber and the child can then inhale this medicine from the device without any need to co-ordinate. This gadget enables young children to use their aerosols more easily and efficiently, as it is a most effective way of getting drug particles deep into the small airways.

NEBULISER  A small machine, either electronic, electrical or manual, which pumps compressed air through a flexible plastic tube to a container holding a liquid bronchodilator. This is connected to a face mask through which the patient inhales the ensuing vaporised medication.

PATHOGENESIS  The mode of development of a disease.

PEAK FLOW METER  This is a simple device for measuring how fast the air can be forced out of the lungs after taking a full breath.

| | |
|---|---|
| PHYSICIAN | A medical doctor other than a surgeon. |
| PLATELET ACTIVATING FACTOR (PAF) | Important in animals and possibly man. Is released by basophils and causes platelets to clump with release of histamines. |
| PNEUMONIA | A lung inflammation, or infection of the alveoli of the lungs caused by any of various agents, such as bacteria or virus. |
| PROGNOSIS | A prediction of the probable course of a disease in an individual and the chances of recovery. |
| PROPHYLACTIC | Protective or preventative medicine. A prophylactic medicine is one which guards against disease. |
| PROSTAGLANDINS | A group of mediators (see MEDIATOR) having various actions on different organs of the body, including some allergic reactions. |
| PROVOCATION TEST | A test carried out to provoke certain symptoms in an individual in order to identify the cause of an allergy, or to test the effectiveness of a drug. |
| PUFFER | A colloquial term referring to small gadgets used to inhale asthma medications, e.g. spinhaler, rotahaler, pressurised aerosol canisters. |
| RECEPTOR SITES | Localised areas of various tissues (cells) where chemical and immunological reactions occur. |
| REGISTRAR | A hospital doctor senior to a houseman and junior to a consultant. |

RESIDENCY — A period of advanced, specialised medical or surgical training at a hospital.

RESIDENT — A person who is serving a residency.

RESPIRATION — Act or process of breathing.

RESPIRATOR — An apparatus for giving artificial respiration.

RHINITIS — Inflammation (infective or allergic) of the mucous membrane of the nose, resulting in a discharge and blockage of the nasal membranes.

ROTAHALER — A small plastic device which, when twisted sharply, breaks open a capsule containing a powdered medication. This may then be inhaled through the mouthpiece of the device.

SALBUTAMOL — A bronchodilator (Ventolin) given by mouth, inhalation as a spray, or by injection. Its action is more prolonged than that of Adrenaline.

SKIN TEST — A means of introducing known allergens to the body to gauge a reaction, by placing a drop of the substance onto the skin and then scratching the area with a pin to ensure absorption. A positive reaction will be shown by a localised area of swelling similar to a sting or nettle rash. These may itch but will not be painful and the swelling should subside between 30 and 60 minutes.

SODIUM CROMOGLYCATE — See INTAL.

SPACER — Smaller than a nebuhaler, but performs a similar function. Its compact size makes it easy to carry in a pocket or a school bag. Like the nebuhaler, the spacer slows the rate at which the drug particles are travelling and reduces their size, so that the impact on the patient's mouth and throat is reduced.

SPECIALIST — See CONSULTANT.

SPINHALER — See ROTAHALER.

SPIROMETER — A device for measuring how much air is forced out of the lungs after a full inspiration. The spirometer can also be used to measure how much air can be driven out after a certain time—usually between three-quarters and one second.

SPORES — Very small particles given off by fungi (see FUNGI), somewhat resembling the pollen of flowers and having a similar function.

STEROIDS (Short for Corticosteroids) — A group of chemical compounds used in the treatment of severe and/or persistent asthma, such as Cortisone and related substances, e.g. Prednisolone. Many steroids occur naturally in the body. Given as tablets, inhalation or injection.

SYMPATHOMIMETICS — A group of substances having varying effects on the body. Some, including Adrenaline, Ephedrine, Salbutamol, are used in asthma because of their prompt bronchodilatory effects.

| | |
|---|---|
| SYSTEMIC | A drug given by mouth or injection which affects the whole body system. |
| THERAPEUTIC | Serving to cure or heal. |
| THERAPY | Treatment by medical or physical means. |
| THORACIC | Of, in, or near the thorax. |
| THORAX | The chest. |
| THRUSH (CANDIDIASIS) | A localised infection caused by a fungus which forms milky-white lesions (sores) on the mouth, lips, throat. |
| TOPICAL | A topical medication has an effect only on the particular part of the body to which it is applied, e.g. an inhaled steroid medication such as Becotide has an effect on the lungs. |
| TRACHEA | Main airway, windpipe. |
| TRIGGER | Something which causes or sets into action. |
| VAPORISER | A machine which changes liquid into vapour. |
| VENTILATOR | An artificial breathing apparatus used to introduce fresh air and drive out foul air (see RESPIRATOR). |
| VENTOLIN | See SALBUTAMOL. |
| VIRULENT | Violent and rapid in its course. |
| VIRUS | Any of a group of ultra-microscopic infective agents that cause various diseases. |
| WHEEZING | To breathe hard with a whistling, breathy sound. |
| WHEEZY BRONCHITIS | A form of asthma, brought on by an infection such as the common cold. |

# Book List

Althea (1982). *I Have Asthma*, Dinosaur Books.

Clark, T.J.H., and Rees, J. (1985). *Practical Management of Asthma*, Martin Dunitz.

Godfrey, S. (1975). *Your Child with Asthma*, Heinemann Health Books.

Jones, R.S. (1976). *Asthma in Children*, Edward Arnold.

Knight, Allan (1981). *Asthma and Hayfever*, Positive Health Guides, Martin Dunitz.

Lane, Donald J., and Storr, Anthony (1979). *Asthma: the Facts*, Oxford University Press.

Milner, A.D. (1984). *Asthma in Childhood*, Churchill Livingstone.

Rackman, K., Thomas, R.V., and Smith, I.J. (1976). *The Child with Asthma*, Invalid Children's Association.

Rapp, D.J., and Frankland, A.W. (1976). *Allergies: Questions and Answers*, Heinemann Health Books.

Rees, J. *ABC of Asthma*, British Medical Association.

An extensive range of pamphlets and booklets is available from The Asthma Society and Friends of the Asthma Research Council, 300 Upper Street, London N1 2XX.

# Index

abnormal chest signs 44
Adcortyl 135
additives 49, 126
adrenal glands 134
air filtration units 122–123
airways 43, 56, 112, 127, 129, 132, 137, 140
allergens 46, 54
allergic asthmatic 47
allergic child 45, 46 *see also* allergy
allergic reaction 46, 56
allergy 122–127, 140
Alps (Swiss) 53, 125
Alupent 50, 51, 59, 129
animal skin 122
antibiotic 44
anxiety 40
aspirin 126
asthma 9, 47, 50, 144
  and age 34, 36–38, 143, 144, 146
  and allergy 45–47, 54, 56, 122–127, 140, 144
  and aspirin 126
  the attack 118–120
  and bronchodilators 28, 50, 51, 59, 128–129
causes of 36–38, 46–47, 53, 56, 109, 111, 114, 122–128, 140–141, 143–144, 147
and a change of air 52, 53
complications 27–28, 36, 42–44, 84–85
control 11, 52, 120, 143
and cramp 64
and coughing 33–35, 40, 43
deaths from 9, 27
emotion as a cause 40, 121, 124, 131–133, 138
and environment 141–142
and the heart 117
and heredity 111–112, 143, 145
and immunisation 148–150
and infection 36–38, 43–44, 101, 107, 109, 140
and the lungs 96, 117
and parties 110
and pets 114–115, 123–125
relaxation exercises 115–116
and school 97–101, 125, 128
and sport 55, 112, 127–128, 131, 144, 145
and steroids 57–58, 96, 134–140, 146

and stress 40, 53, 132, 141
symptoms 10, 27, 33–39, 43–44, 47, 103, 118–120
and travel 117, 150
and wind instruments 115
and yoga 115
Asthma Society and Friends of the Asthma Research Council 12, 151–153
attacks, Sara 10, 22–30, 39, 59, 73–76, 81–87, 90–93, 95

Beclomethasone 134
Becotide 51, 52, 57, 58, 97, 129–131, 150
bedding 126
bedroom 125–126
Berotec 129
Betamethasone 134
Betnelan 134
Betnesol 134
Bextasol 129, 131, 150
'blanket' treatment 97
breast feeding 144
breath control 115, 145
Bricanyl 129, 131
bronchiolitis 140
Bronchodil 129
bronchodilator 28, 50, 51, 59, 128–129

candidiasis see thrush
carpet 47, 122, 126
cats 125
causes of asthma 36–38, 46–47, 53, 56, 109, 111, 114, 122–128, 140–141, 143–144, 147
cavity-wall insulation 147

Celestone 134
central heating 147
Cetacort 134
change of air 52, 53
chest consultant 10, 35
childish wheezing 36, 37, 38, 41
cigarette smoke 122, 141
cleaning 126
cleaning agents 122
clothing 117, 123
Cobutolin 129
Codelcortone 134
Codelsol 134
cold winds 56, 98
collapse 43, 44, 103
colourings 126
complications 27–28, 36, 42–44, 84–85
control 11, 52, 120, 143
Cortate 134
Cortelan 134
Cortex 134
Cortisab 134
Cortisone 134
Cortisyl 134
Cortone 134
coughing 33–35, 40, 43, 46, 49, 53, 61
cramp 64
cyanosis 27–28, 36, 84–85

damp 55, 56, 141
Decasdron 134
Decortisyl 134
Delta-Cortef 134
Deltacortone 134
Delta-Cortril 134
Deltastab 134

Deltasolone 134
Depo-Medrone 134
desensitising injections 127
detergents *see* cleaning agents
Dexacortisyl 134
Dexamethasone 134
Dexone 134
Di-Adreson 134
diet *see* exclusion diet
dog 114–115, 123
dust 56, 122

eczema 141, 143, 148–150
Efcortelan 134
Efcortisol 134
Eldecort 134
emotions 40, 121, 124, 131–133, 138 *see also* stress
environment 53, 141–142
exercise-induced asthma 55, 127–128
exercises 115–116
exclusion diet 50
Exirel 129
explanations 110–111

face mask 48, 49
family problems 35, 121–122, 124, 133
feathers 122
  birds 123
Fenoterol 129
fish 124
food and drink 49–50, 126, 143
freezer
  mite control 126
fumes 122
fungi 56
fur 122, 124

guilt 107–108
goat's milk 143

hair *see* fur
Haldrate 134
hay fever 53, 147
heart 117
heredity 111–112, 143, 145
high altitudes 142
house dust allergy 56, 122
house dust mite 47, 122, 125, 142
household dust 56, 122, 125–126
humidifiers 123
humidity 55
Hydrocortisab 134
Hydrocortisone 134
Hydrocortone 134
hypnotism 142
hysterics *see* emotions

immunisation 148–150
infection 36–38, 41, 140
inhalers 128–131, 147
  correct use of 136–137
  dangers of 111
Intal (Sodium Cromoglycate) 48, 50–52, 57, 97, 129, 131
ionisers 122–123

Kenalog 135
Kenalone 135

late signs 28
Ledercort 135
Lederspan 135
lethargy 22, 49
lungs 96, 117

measles *see* immunisation
Medic-Alert bracelet 136
medications
   artificial colouring 126
   bronchodilators 128–129
   corticosteroids      129–130,
      134–140
   explanations 121
   Sodium Cromoglycate (Intal)
      129
   timetables 102
   tooth decay 126
Medihaler-Iso 129
Medro-Cortex 134
Medrol 134
Medrone 134
Methyl-Prednisolone 134
Meticortelone 134
Metilar 134
migraine 143
mites *see* house dust mite
moon face 72, 139
mould 55, 56, 122
mucus 43–44

nebuhaler 130
nebuliser 48, 49, 69, 89, 93, 95,
      97, 117, 118

Oradexon 134
Orciprenaline 129
organisations 151–154
   overseas 153–154

pain 64, 103
Paramethasone 134
peak flow meters 112
personality
   asthmatic 121, 131–133

pets 114–115, 123–125
Phyllocontin *see* Theophylin
physiotherapy 44
Pirbuterol 129
plug
   mucus 43–44
pneumonia 42–44
Polar regions 125
pollen 55–56, 122
precautions 47
Precortisyl 134
Prednesol 134
Prednisolone 134
Prelone 134
preventative treatment 127,
      129, 137
prophylactic treatment *see* pre-
      ventative treatment
Pulmadil 129
puffer 102
Pulmicort 130, 150

questions and answers 141–150

relaxation exercises 115–116
Reproterol 129
research 11, 151
rotahaler 51, 97

Salbulin 129
Salbutamol 129
saliva 122, 124
school
   absence from 100
   change of 99
   check list 101
   problems 98
   solutions 99–101, 125, 128

seasonal changes 55 *see also* thunderstorms
Sintisone 134
skin tests 46, 70, 144
Slo-Phyllin *see* Theophylin
Sodium Cromoglycate (Intal) 48, 129
soft toys 126
Solu-Cortef 134
Solu-Medrone 134
spacer 130
spinhaler *see* rotahaler
spores 55
sports 128, 131, 144, 145
steroids 57–58, 96, 134–140, 146
  side effects 72, 138–140
  tablets, Sara 71
stress 40, 53, 132, 141
stomach ache *see* cramp
swimming 112
Switzerland 53, 142
symptoms 10, 27, 33–39, 43–44, 47, 103, 118–120
systemic steroids 136

tantrums *see* emotions
Terbutaline 129
tests
  airways 112
  skin tests 46, 70, 144
Theophylin 89, 97, 128
thunderstorms 108–110
thrush 138
topical steroids 136
travel 117, 150
Triamacin 135
Triamcinolone 135
trigger 47, 96

Ventolin 28, 59, 65, 68, 95, 129, 131
  side effects 144

weight gain 72, 138
wheezing 9, 36–38, 53, 59, 64, 96, 127–131, 140
wheezy bronchitis 36–38 *see also* childish wheezing
whooping cough 148–150

yoga 115